Trauma and Birth

Our book aims to provide those working in the maternity services, including those in general practices, with an understanding of what it means to be on the receiving end of care. Together with a description of various types of traumatic birth, we explain some of the reasons why women vary in terms of how traumatised they are by their birth experience. We provide information, encouragement and support for maternity staff to help them lessen the incidence of birth trauma, and to develop the confidence to help women when birth trauma does occur.

The authors are a senior counsellor and an obstetrician, each with a long experience of helping women who have had difficult births. The approach of each to the subject is different but complementary. The book covers the psychological and emotional aspects of traumatic birth as well as the medical issues and includes a section on the effect of traumatic birth on the staff themselves.

The market for this book is practising midwives and obstetricians, who by understanding the prevalence of traumatic birth and some of its causes can contribute to its reduction. Those in their training years will find it helpful at the outset of their practice. It will also be of interest to general practitioners, health visitors and counsellors.

Sheila Broderick qualified as a Social Worker in 1977. She initially worked at a therapeutic community for people with drug addiction. She then worked for Greenwich Mind, mental health charity, before she left to work at University Lewisham Hospital as a Women's Health Counsellor. Her work at the hospital was always woman-centred, with kindness, support and an acknowledgement of each person's uniqueness at its heart. When she retired in 2013 she was Senior Women's Health Counsellor.

Ruth Cochrane has been a Consultant Obstetrician and Gynaecologist since 1997. She is a busy generalist and is regularly to be found on the labour ward. She is particularly interested in high-risk obstetrics, major benign gynaecological surgery, the management of perinatal loss and undergraduate education. She runs a postnatal debrief clinic for women and their partners who have had traumatic births.

Trauma and Birth

A Handbook for Maternity Staff

Sheila Broderick and Ruth Cochrane

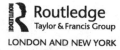
Routledge
Taylor & Francis Group

LONDON AND NEW YORK

First published 2021
by Routledge
2 Park Square, Milton Park, Abingdon, Oxon OX14 4RN

and by Routledge
52 Vanderbilt Avenue, New York, NY 10017

Routledge is an imprint of the Taylor & Francis Group, an informa business

British Library Cataloguing-in-Publication Data
A catalogue record for this book is available from the British Library

Library of Congress Cataloging-in-Publication Data
A catalog record for this book has been requested

ISBN: 978-0-367-42040-6 (hbk)
ISBN: 978-0-367-51346-7 (pbk)
ISBN: 978-0-367-81751-0 (ebk)

Typeset in Bembo
by Apex CoVantage, LLC

Contents

Acknowledgements

We want to acknowledge all the women who have needed our support after experiencing a traumatic birth. They have contributed to the writing of this book, either by trusting us with their experiences through our work or by telling us their stories explicitly for the purpose of this book.

We also want to acknowledge all our colleagues who work within the maternity services. In writing this book we have become even more aware of how being a compassionate, caring health worker can be exciting and exhilarating but can also be traumatising.

Introduction

We have worked as a consultant obstetrician and a senior women's health counsellor (nearly 20 years for Sheila and over 23 years and counting for Ruth) in a busy NHS hospital in South East London. Through our individual and joint work with pregnant and postpartum women, their partners and families, we realised that there needed to be a book for staff about traumatic birth: a book that addresses the concerns women have raised with us, many of which are hidden until they are given the opportunity to 'see the light of day'. When gathering material for the book and looking beyond our own interactions with women, we realised that what we had suspected was indeed true, that traumatic births are very common and that women are left suffering, shocked and upset.

Traumatic birth is a current and on-going concern in the United Kingdom, both at a national and regional level. The Birth Trauma Association states that as many as a third of women report their birth experience as being traumatic. One in 25 women will go on to be diagnosed as having posttraumatic stress disorder (PTSD) as a result of their birth experience. It is certainly an issue for women. One has only to do an internet search for traumatic birth to find many, many stories of women's feelings of alienation and distress during their labour and birth experience. These statistics are really important and show that practices need to change to bring about a reduction in the numbers. The significance of a traumatic birth cannot and should not be underestimated.

There are two dominant reasons given as the causes of traumatic birth: unnecessary medical interventions and the lack of a relationship with the caregiver. We attempt to address aspects of both of these and the interaction between the two. What a woman might call unnecessary won't always tally with what an obstetrician thinks. We will try to talk about the gap, or gulf, between what women believe and what obstetricians think they know, which may in itself be different from the opinion of midwives. This is apparent when talking about birth plans, which we discuss in one of our chapters.

We look at medical interventions during labour, including instrumental delivery, tears, Caesarean sections and other surgical procedures. Additionally, we observe the potential traumatic impact of anaesthesia during labour and delivery and of being in an intensive care unit.

Mental health is an important consideration for all of us and there are specific issues relating to birth that affect our mental health (not the least the impact that traumatic birth has on mental wellbeing) and we have devoted a chapter to this topic.

There is a distinct difference between what is deemed a complicated birth and an uncomplicated birth. The complicated one is likely to be recognised by staff as potentially involving or causing trauma, whilst the uncomplicated one is not. The difference is illustrated in the chapter regarding the experience of traumatic birth. It is interesting that sometimes a birth that has been dramatic to medical staff and therefore recognised as potentially traumatic is not always perceived to be by the mother. More than one patient who has 'been through the mill' has reported that she did not understand why lots of staff members were coming to her after the birth and saying 'You have had a bad time'. It may be that because the obstetric complications required interventions, the woman got a particular kind of care and felt looked after despite needing additional recovery time, and so she herself was not traumatised. This is not to say that she should not be offered support and help to understand what happened to make her birth complicated. This illustrates to some extent just how differently individuals react. The causes of trauma and the experience of trauma differ from one person to another. Ruth recounts that in one recovery room where she worked there was a notice which read 'Pain is what the patient says it is'. Pain is personal and cannot be determined from the outside. The same is true of trauma. There should *never* be any judgements or assumptions made about the experience or degree of trauma experienced by individuals; it may well be that judgements and assumptions contributed to the trauma in the first instance.

In the chapter on person-centred care we cover some of the issues regarding the need for continuity of care and the need for empowering pregnant and labouring women through establishing an equal relationship with caregivers. We try to give an insight into what it means to be a 'patient' and point out that whether staff realise it or not, they are often in a position of power. We recognise that many workers do not feel powerful and that it is up to managers to create a culture of care and regard for staff to enable them to be better caregivers.

We have included a chapter on tears. These are a source of trauma for some women, either because the care they received was inadequate and a tear occurred as a result, or because they have not received the appropriate aftercare.

This book is primarily about raising the awareness of the occurrence of traumatic birth and its frequency for staff working in hospital maternity units, community clinics and GP practices. Treatment of PTSD and postnatal depression are beyond our scope and speciality and we have not addressed these ailments specifically in our book. However, it is worth noting that it is not uncommon for traumatic birth to be misdiagnosed as postnatal depression. It would be helpful if GPs and health visitors were able to ask a woman about her birth experience if they suspected that she was depressed after giving birth.

As an obstetrician and a counsellor another aspect of our work has been pregnancy loss. We have looked after women who were bereaved by early and late miscarriage, stillbirths and neonatal deaths. We have not included their trauma in this book as we have covered it in an earlier publication (Broderick & Cochrane 2013). Our observation would be that bereaved women and their partners did not report the actual birth of their baby to be traumatic *other* than when the care was not as it should have been. When the care was less than good, their grief and loss was made worse by their experience. Such was the insult and injury caused by the lack of care that their ability to grieve was impaired.

Lack of regard and care for their individual circumstances creates similar feelings to those women and partners who are traumatised whilst having a live baby. The distress caused is intermingled with their feelings of loss but the questions of 'why me?' and the feelings of powerlessness and of being inconsequential are experienced by women in both situations. They also share the need to have an opportunity to have a debrief with a senior obstetrician or midwife who can understand their experience and who can also help them with the next pregnancy should they want to be pregnant again. We have included chapters on debrief and managing the next delivery. We want to encourage staff to learn about how useful it is for people to be understood and cared for after a traumatic birth, and about how whilst not being able to alter the suffering at the time of birth we can help women and their birth partners heal some of their distress.

It is important to be aware of the issue of language, and how it is used within medical settings. Does it lead staff consciously or unconsciously to contribute to creating trauma? For example, is a pregnant woman from the moment of her first visit to a medical setting automatically a patient? What does being a patient mean? Does being a patient indicate passivity? Community midwives where we work tend not to refer to pregnant women as patients, instead calling them clients. Does being referred to as a pregnant woman or a client, rather than a patient, lessen the likelihood of a traumatic birth? What does being in labour mean to women as opposed to medical personnel? It is not unusual that women will perceive themselves as being in labour for 24 or 48 hours whilst their notes will indicate that they were in labour for 8 or 12 hours. This is discussed in the chapters on prolonged labour and instrumental delivery.

What does an emergency mean? Emergency Caesarean sections have three categories within a hospital setting and action is taken by staff according to the category, but it is rare that patients understand this. As a result, women who are not in the most urgent category can be traumatised because they were expecting their procedure to happen much more quickly than it did. Alternatively, those who are in the most critical category often feel powerless, because things start happening to them very quickly and they often feel excluded from the decisions made – this may well be despite having to sign a consent form. This is discussed further in the chapter on Caesarean sections and other surgical interventions.

We conclude with a chapter regarding the trauma experienced by staff. We want to acknowledge how challenging maternity care can be and that workers in this field are not immune to facing stress as a consequence of their daily work. This is a branch of health-care that is enormously rewarding but which comes with its own versions of difficulty, sadness and challenge. As we were writing this final chapter, we became aware of how vital it is to acknowledge the cost of being a conscientious worker within the caring professions and in particular in obstetrics. There is a section within the chapter that explores various scenarios where something goes wrong in labour in which we have used the term 'bad', recognising that the experience has been traumatic for everyone involved in the birth. Trauma and birth can go together for the woman having the baby and also for the staff who are doing their best to help her: that is why we wrote this book.

Reference

Broderick S, Cochrane R. *Perinatal loss: A handbook for working with women and their families.* London: Radcliffe, 2013.

1　The experience of traumatic birth

Experiencing a traumatic birth can have a devastating effect on a mother and a marked effect on her nearest and dearest. One of the consequences of this can be that the woman feels isolated and misunderstood. Additionally, she may feel especially estranged from her baby. This estrangement only compounds the horrible way she feels. It is highly likely that she will not have been expecting to have to cope with either or both of the physical and emotional assaults on her being that a traumatic birth can bring.

Many women post-delivery are desperately unhappy because of their birth experience. This misery is regardless of whether the trauma was due to a medical intervention, an emergency or an apparently (as deemed by the obstetricians) uncomplicated labour.

The Birth Trauma Association states

> Birth trauma is a shorthand phrase for post-traumatic stress disorder (PTSD) after childbirth. We also use it for women who have some symptoms of PTSD, but not enough for a full diagnosis.
>
> PTSD was first identified amongst soldiers returning from the Vietnam War, and most people still think of it as a condition experienced by soldiers. In fact, PTSD can follow any traumatic event – such as being in a car accident, being sexually abused or having a very difficult birth. It can also happen to people who have witnessed a traumatic event, so people who have seen someone else violently killed, for example, often experience PTSD. This is why some partners, and even midwives, experience PTSD after seeing a traumatic birth.
>
> In most cases, what makes birth traumatic is the fear that you or your baby are going to die. We very often see birth trauma in women who have lost a lot of blood, for example, or who had to have an emergency caesarean because their baby's heart-rate suddenly dipped.

Symptoms of birth trauma (postnatal PTSD)

There are four main symptoms:

- Re-experiencing the traumatic event through flashbacks, nightmares or intrusive memories. These make you feel distressed and panicky.
- Avoiding anything that reminds you of the trauma. This can mean refusing to walk past the hospital where you gave birth, or avoiding meeting other women with new babies.
- Feeling hypervigilant: this means that you are constantly alert, irritable and jumpy. You worry that something terrible is going to happen to your baby.

- Feeling low and unhappy ('negative cognition' in the medical jargon). You may feel guilty and blame yourself for your traumatic birth. You may have difficulty remembering parts of your birth experience.

Not everyone who has had a traumatic experience suffers from PTSD, but many do. It's a completely normal response, and not a sign of weakness. It is also involuntary: brain scans show a difference between the brains of people with PTSD and those without. PTSD is not something that can be cured by 'pulling yourself together' or 'focusing on the positive', despite what other people tell you.

Who gets birth trauma?

Some women experience events during childbirth (as well as in pregnancy or immediately after birth) that would traumatise any normal person. For other women, it is not always the sensational or dramatic events that trigger childbirth trauma but other factors such as loss of control, loss of dignity, the hostile attitudes of the people around them, feelings of not being heard or the absence of informed consent to medical procedures. Some of the reasons for trauma given by the Birth Trauma Association are listed below:

- Lengthy labour or short and very painful labour
- Induction
- Poor pain relief
- Feelings of loss of control
- High levels of medical intervention
- Forceps births
- Emergency caesarean section
- Impersonal treatment or problems with staff attitudes
- Not being listened to
- Lack of information or explanation
- Lack of privacy and dignity
- Fear for baby's safety
- Stillbirth
- Birth of a baby with a disability resulting from a traumatic birth
- Baby's stay in the special care baby unit or neonatal intensive care unit
- Poor postnatal care
- Previous trauma (for example, in childhood, with a previous birth or domestic violence)

Finally, people who witness their partner's traumatic childbirth experience may also feel traumatised as a result.

(Birth Trauma Association)

Experiences of a traumatic birth

One woman I met was a first-time mother who had a CS following a protracted labour. Whilst in the recovery ward it became clear to staff that she was losing blood. She then needed to go back to theatre for an emergency procedure to stem the blood. The procedure was successful and she was no longer in danger. She was taken to the Intensive Care Unit to recover. She spent several days there.

Her experience of what happened was extremely overwhelming and when I met her after six months, she was struggling to make sense of why she felt so bad. She was unable to believe that she was a good mother, which was understandably very hard for her.

Together we began to unravel her experience of giving birth and it became clear that she did not understand exactly what had happened and why they did in the way that they did. She needed a debrief with an experienced clinician who could explain what happened from an obstetric point of view and who could also understand her version of events. The latter is crucially important in the case of a debrief. It is not enough to explain to the patient what happened and why without being prepared to *include* and *acknowledge* the perspective of the mother and often her partner. The senior practitioner needs to be prepared to alter their version (which will often be a written one) after listening to the experience of the mother and her birth partner. This can be a painstaking consultation but really, really worth doing, as it can sometimes lift the veil of confusion that has blighted the woman's experience of birth. Without this level of empathy, you will be in danger of causing additional injury and leave her more isolated.

The reaction to a traumatic birth and its aftermath is individual and this needs to be respected by all those who encounter someone in the midst of the trauma. It is essential that her thoughts, feelings and reactions are not dismissed with a quick retort or comment. You are dealing with someone whose self-image is likely to have been shaken beyond her wildest imagination.

Going back to the woman mentioned above, the debrief was extremely useful, as she and her partner were able to ask the questions they had been pondering over for six months. She was able to ask if her life was ever in danger. A significant moment for her was when she went to theatre for the emergency operation to stem the blood loss, one of the medical staff told her that her family had been called, as was normal in these circumstances. Whatever the staff member meant by that comment, what she heard was that she was in danger of losing her life and she underwent the anaesthetic thinking that she had just given birth to her son and that she might never see him or her husband again. This is an example of what we refer to in our introduction: that the words said at any time, let alone at moments of crisis, have a huge impact.

She did not die but woke up in the Intensive Care Unit. This experience of Intensive Care is covered in another chapter; sufficient to say here that it is not easy to find yourself waking up in a place which is associated with being extremely ill or with a life-threatening condition. One of her thoughts was 'how did I end up here when I came in to give birth to my son?'

The separation from her son had a profound effect on her and she missed the first days of his life. This was justifiably difficult for her – especially when she will have heard all about skin-to-skin contact being essential in establishing mother and baby bonding. She went home as soon as she could as she wanted to get away from the hospital environment. What had not been explained to her was that, given what she had been through, she was likely to feel poorly for quite some time. Without this knowledge she was left with her own coping mechanisms to manage the trauma she had experienced. It is important to understand that without appropriate explanation, someone who goes from walking into hospital as a healthy person and who ends up in Intensive Care will not really have any comprehension as why they feel so physically, emotionally and sometimes psychologically depleted and feeling ill for such a long time.

As a means of understanding their experience, different people have diverse ways of managing. Some will devour television programmes covering medical emergencies, trying to see if other people cope in the way they did. Others will avoid any mention of hospitals and switch off the television at the mere mention of medical emergencies, as they do not want any reminder of their trauma. Once home, the mother expected to feel well and she did not understand why she was so tired and weak. She did manage to establish breastfeeding and fed her baby whenever he needed. She also had him close by her. She had a supportive husband and he looked after her well, but it was also very challenging for him to understand the changes in his wife.

Six months later she felt she had physically improved but she was still feeling extremely bad because she felt she had let her son down and that she had been a 'bad' mother. Part of our work together was helping her to separate her feelings of failure from the fact that she *had* been a good mother. Her feelings of failure were due to the fact that she had not experienced the warmth of connection between herself and her son that she expected to have. This lack of feeling of a connection was profound for her and not something she could ever regain. She did begin to feel close to her son but she had to grieve for the loss of closeness during the first few months. She also needed help to see that her son would not necessarily feel the same kind of loss as her: he had the closeness he needed.

One of the consequences of her trauma was that she did not want to interact with people as she had previously. This was sometimes a cause of tension between her and her partner. Her resources were severely diminished and she needed help to gradually rebuild these. The way that she did this was to only do things that were within her scope of capability at any one particular time. Prior to the trauma she had been highly efficient, and losing the ability to live like this was very challenging for her. It is not an understatement to say she did not recognise herself and she did not understand how this loss had happened. Some of the healing work we did was for her to give herself permission to consciously take control and to only do what was right for her. Learning 'to walk (again) before she could run' was frustrating for her and her family; they too had expectations of her being as she had been. Gradually as she took her time to believe in her reality, albeit a reality she would have much preferred not to have, she began to recognise herself again. The impact of her trauma continued despite her recovery. Two years after the birth of her son she was not at all sure if she wanted to have another baby. Her fear of something similar happening was so great that she could not contemplate another pregnancy.

The emotional aftermath of being in Intensive Care and how long it may take to begin to recover physically, let alone emotionally, needs to be understood by the patient, her family and all those who are looking after her: labour ward staff, community staff and GPs to mention a few. The experience of the woman described above would probably always have been challenging and traumatic but several interventions at an earlier stage could have helped her and her family enormously. Had she and her husband been appropriately informed prior to leaving the hospital, then they would have had some idea of what to expect. It is the equivalent of being 'forewarned is forearmed'. Had she been helped to understand the length of time it would take her to recover physically, let alone emotionally, she would have had an explanation for her exhaustion. She would not have had to wait until she saw her obstetric consultant six months later who confirmed that her postnatal experience was to be expected and normal, given what she had been through. She would not have needed to have struggled without help from a counsellor to begin to make sense of the impact of her trauma. It is terrible to think that oversights like this happen daily.

The failure to notice the needs of women and their partners condemns them to isolation and further trauma. Empathy, understanding and the ability to relate is not high-tech.

It does not require investment in expensive instruments, but the effects are as dramatic as any technical procedure.

We cannot stress enough the importance of developing a trusting relationship with pregnant and labouring women. There were 657,076 live births in England and Wales in 2018. If one-third of the mothers experienced trauma, some of which were due to a lack of a relationship with their caregivers (one of the major causes for traumatic birth), it means that a large number of these nearly 220,000 women could have avoided suffering at the crucial time of birth and the postnatal period.

Providing good care

An example of anticipating a traumatic reaction was described by one woman I talked to as a result of research for this book. The birth of her child was long and protracted, and she ended up with an emergency Caesarean section. Her partner witnessed the harrowing events that led up to the arrival of their baby. The mother did not initially feel that she had experienced any trauma and was to some extent perplexed by the reaction of staff who told her that she had. Before she and her partner left the hospital, she was given the name and telephone number of whom to contact should she begin to experience any symptoms of trauma. Within a number of weeks, she realised she did need to understand more about the circumstances of her experience and that her partner also needed to be included as she, too, had been through an ordeal. Their request for an appointment was acknowledged in an appropriate time frame. They met with an experienced midwife, in a room away from the maternity service. From the outset of the meeting they were made to feel that they and their experience were at the heart of the consultation. The debrief lasted 4 hours, which might seem excessive to some but it was worth every moment. As a result, both parents understood exactly what had happened from an obstetric viewpoint, and why certain decisions were made. Additionally, they were able to describe their individual reactions and responses to what had happened. The investment made by that particular hospital in their care probably saved the NHS at lot of money, as any longer lasting effects of trauma did not need to be treated by medication and visits to a GP. The hospital she attended was geared up for helping women who have a traumatic birth and had invested the necessary time and appropriate training for staff to offer continued care beyond the labour ward.

It should be a requirement that medical personnel appreciate that patients' reactions to their experience varies greatly. We have known women who, from an obstetric point of view, have had horrendous births and who then find themselves to be the focus of much staff attention. The patient is surprised by the number of staff who come to them and tell them what a hard time they have had and keep asking how they are. It is certainly our experience that some patients do not perceive themselves as traumatised. This does not mean that they should not be offered a debrief and given appropriate information as to what to expect of themselves during their recovery. This information should include what to do should they begin to struggle to make sense of their experience at some point in the future. Conversely, there are many women who are regarded as having a routine or not particularly stressful labour, but who from their own point of view have had a traumatic birth.

We worked with a patient who had retained placenta and a postpartum haemorrhage. The correct obstetric procedures were carried out, i.e. she went to theatre to have her placenta removed and a blood transfusion. She then went to the postnatal ward. This patient's experience was not deemed to be anything out of the ordinary as she was looked after according to the procedures that exist to deal with what happened at the birth. For the patient, however, the experience of needing to go to theatre and having lost so much blood shook her to the core. She loved her daughter and she did not doubt that she had been a good mother. However, it was very difficult for her to believe that anyone else could look after her daughter well.

With the help of counselling she was able to make sense of her feelings. In the debrief it was really particularly important for her to know if her life had ever been in danger. The response was that she was never likely to die because she was in the right place with the right people, i.e. her blood loss was dealt with appropriately. Had she been in the wrong place then she could well have been in danger. This clarification really helped her: she seemed able to regain her trust in life.

Within an obstetric department there will be a 'scale' of what is acceptable in relation to birth. Hospital staff are (or should be) geared up to deal with complications in labour because they are trained for just such events. Only the cases with complications will require scrutiny as to what occurred and what, if anything, went wrong, but what is routine within a hospital will not necessarily be anything like ordinary to many patients.

What is the experience like for women who will have been perceived to have had a routine birth?

This category of women can include women who, for all intents and purposes, had an ordinary, uncomplicated labour, and also covers women who have been in a High Dependency Unit. As said earlier, some complications in labour can be fairly normal and therefore staff may not always recognise that the woman is experiencing difficulty in coping with what for her is 'something wrong or frightening'. She can therefore be confused as to why (in contrast to the obstetric staff's reaction to a complicated event) no one is paying her attention or why, when she exhibits symptoms of distress, she is given short shrift.

We know of a woman who had a third-degree tear and who on the postnatal ward was mortified to find that she had lost control of her bowels. Until she had a debrief, which did not take place until some considerable time after birth, no one had told her that due to her injury she would have been given medication to loosen her bowels to avoid strain and thereby further damage. If she had known that a degree of incontinence was normal, then her considerable distress would have been avoided altogether.

This woman's labour had been prolonged and complicated by the fact that her baby was in the 'back to back' position. This fact was not realised for some considerable time into her labour. Without this information she was left feeling a failure as all her efforts felt as if they were in vain. Her birth partner, her husband, found refuge in the machinery that was present in the room, i.e. he did not know how to cope with a long, protracted labour either. His wife was hurt by his behaviour and it took her a long time to forgive his inattention to her. Had the reason for the slow progress been discovered and explained sooner, both parents could have been helped and guided through the complicated birth of their son. Back-to-back or occipito-posterior (OP) positions are not rare but do need staff to understand how women are likely to feel and to know how they might be helped. This will include trying different positions in labour, offering different types of pain relief, and being sympathetic if none of those measures make a difference to the baby's position.

In attempt to mitigate trauma at birth we conclude by examining the list of causes of traumatic birth provided by the Birth Trauma Association: it is fair to say that some of the causes given are unavoidable and some are not.

The length of labour is to some degree beyond anyone's control, but an unnecessarily prolonged birth is an indication of lack of individual care.

Poor pain relief is inexcusable. Taking care of labouring women has to include making her as comfortable as possible and responding to her needs as they change during labour.

Induction, forceps delivery, high levels of medical intervention, emergency Caesarean section and a baby going to a neonatal unit may be necessary during any delivery. The way that any of these interventions is handled by those performing them can contribute to a mother's understanding and ability to deal with the unexpected. If interventions are handled badly it is understandable that trauma occurs. Trauma may also occur if the mother had very clear thoughts about how her labour would go and interventions were not part of her plans.

Stillbirth and a baby born with a disability resulting from a traumatic birth have huge impacts both for the parents and staff involved. Investigations will need to take place and parents offered appropriate, honest responses to their questions and heartache.

Not being listened to, lack of privacy and dignity, lack of information or explanation, impersonal treatment or problems with staff attitudes are issues which could be instantly remedied if person-centred care is at the heart of maternity services. Staff attitudes to any patient have been shown to make a huge difference to the good or the bad. Good post-natal care is crucial to women after giving birth, both on the postnatal ward and at home. Midwives looking after women after birth have huge opportunities to relate to women and all their concerns and worries; they can increase confidence or they can make women feel inadequate.

Fear for the baby's safety and previous trauma may be hidden from staff. It is our contention that if a trusting relationship is established, women may well confide in their midwife or doctor. A joint birth plan can be created to anticipate and manage potential trauma prior to birth.

It is unlikely that all traumatic births can be avoided: the 'ingredients' that contribute to the suffering and pain are too subjective for all traumatic births to be eradicated. That said, it is clear that a significant number of traumatic births could be mitigated by the commitment to person-centred care.

Reference

www.birthtraumaassociation.org.uk

2 Person-centred care

Our use of the word *patient* is not in any way to be interpreted to mean that we are adopting a medical model of care. We will use *patient*, as well as *woman, mother, father* and *partner*, as a description for people who are on the receiving end of care from maternity staff. When we are discussing person–centred care, we do at times substitute *patient* for *person* to avoid too much repetition.

Those in receipt of care or treatment should be equal and vital participants in their own experiences. This unfortunately is not always the case. This chapter is an attempt to aid maternity staff to begin to think about what it means to be a patient and how hidden or more obvious power dynamics contribute to undermining individuals. That said, we acknowledge that institutions, particularly hierarchical ones, by their very nature also undermine individual staff members' feelings of power.

As a society, and indeed as human beings, we are challenged by dealing with difference. Many of the problems that exist in relation to equality and inequality are founded on a tendency to categorise ourselves in a hierarchical manner, hierarchical meaning that those with more power believe they are superior.

Martin Buber, a German theologist writing in 1923, proposed that there is a different way of relating. He perceived human beings as relating to the world in two ways, either *I-Thou* or *I-It*. The former is one of equality: *I-Thou* is respectful of the relation between two beings. The latter, the *I-It* relation, is a way of relating which means distancing oneself from the other (the *It*). In the *I-Thou* relationship, human beings acknowledge the connection of beingness. Human beings do not see each other as having separate, superior individuality, but rather that any dialogue between them respects and acknowledges each other's whole being. With the *I-It* relationship, human beings perceive each other as consisting of an individual, separate quality, and see themselves as belonging to a world which consists of things. *I-Thou* is a relationship of mutual respect and interchange, whilst *I-It* is a relationship of disconnection and dispassion.

Being in need of care in a medical setting does not make one less than the person offering the care. It is an opportunity to engage in the *I-Thou* relationship as proposed by Martin Buber.

One of the major reasons given as to why women experience childbirth–related PTSD is that they do not feel treated well and appropriately by their care providers. Feeling mistreated by care providers is a powerful indication that traumatised women have not felt equal partners in the process of their labour and giving birth; it means that the care a woman received was highly likely not to have been centred on her, i.e. she did not experience herself as receiving person–centred care. In other words, she was not part of the *I-Thou* relationship.

A relationship based on equality within health care is known as person-centred care. Person-centred care is different from a more conventional model, which views the patient as a passive participant of medical care. Rather than the outdated model where a health professional makes recommendations to a patient, the person-centred care model includes the patient and their relatives in making joint decisions and agreements about their care regarding plans and treatments. Person-centred care is a partnership between the health care professionals, the patient and their relatives.

Care which puts the person at the heart of any treatment should, of course, be given to all patients, including pregnant and labouring women. From listening to patients and researching material for this book it is clear that a lack of person-centred care, or the *I-Thou* relationship, has frequently caused the 'injury' which contributes to a traumatic birth.

What do we mean by person-centred care?

Person-centred care has many definitions but a well-accepted one is offered by the Institute of Medicine (www.kingsfund.org.uk): 'providing care that is respectful of and responsive to individual patient preferences, needs, and values and ensuring that patient values guide all clinical decisions. In today's NHS it has come to mean putting the patient and their experience at the heart of quality improvement. Person-centred care is one aspect of health care quality, as important as care being safe, clinically effective, timely and equitable'.

Patient-centred care is multi-dimensional: it encompasses all aspects of how services are delivered to patients. The Institute of Medicine offers this list:

* Compassion, empathy and responsiveness to needs, values and expressed preferences
* Emotional support, relieving fear and anxiety
* Coordination and integration
* Physical comfort
* Involvement of family and friends
* Information, communication and education

Enabling provision of person-centred care requires that staff are supported and that they in turn experience equal respect and regard from their managers and institutions as is being required of them.

Jocelyn Cornwell (2017), chief executive of the Point of Care Foundation, writes in her guest blog for the Kings Fund: 'Members of the executive team would not leave the quality of relational care to chance but would see their role as identifying and dismantling systemic obstacles to good care. They would aim to protect and increase the time that frontline staff spend with patients, by reducing the administrative load and culling top-down demands for information. Accepting that surveys have their limitations; they would seek multiple sources of intelligence about the quality of care and listen to the views and opinions of patients and staff'.

Offering patient-centred care can initially appear to be demanding, but the benefits will be evident once patient and staff satisfaction begins to be taken into account. People working within the health profession do so because they want to provide care. It is often systems which prevent them from providing that care. At its most basic level, person-centred care requires changes in the structure. For example, it requires changes in hospital procedures: that there is recognition of patients' reality rather than running services that suit the organisation. Some changes are already happening, e.g. providing appointments at times other than between 9am and 5pm for those who work. It could mean rethinking the way resources are used. Most of all it means a change in the way caregivers *relate* to patients. It requires that medical personnel and all others who meet patients (e.g. receptionists, porters) understand what it is like to be on the receiving end of care. Equipped with that knowledge, staff are able to include kindness, understanding and empathy as essential aspects of their caregiving as well as 'hands-on' care.

The stated vision of the Point of Care Foundation is 'radical improvement in the way we care and are cared for'; their mission 'is to humanise healthcare. We achieve this by working to improve patients' experience of care and increase support for staff who work with them'.

The Collins dictionary definition of humanise is 'to make or become more humane'. It is too easy to be overcome by internal and external pressures which make us forget that we ourselves and those we are looking after are human beings. If health care is to be humanised then we must first examine what it means to be a patient and to attempt to understand the plethora of thoughts and feelings experienced before, during and after treatment.

What does it mean to be dependent on someone else for the quality of care you receive? Finding yourself needing to visit a doctor, midwife or nurse is often a cause of stress for many people, certainly until they are able to form a relationship based on trust, if they are ever able to do so. However, lots of patients report that they never see the same person twice, so they have to deal with each new encounter hoping they will be treated well.

A visit to a GP or hospital can be anxiety-provoking. Even finding the place of the appointment within a hospital can be daunting. Usually hospitals appear to be huge, with lots of signs and corridors. Finding the correct department and then approaching the reception desk with no idea of the system operating there can be very off-putting. As patients we are completely dependent on whom we meet; whether the health care professional is kind, understanding and interested in us or brusque, impatient or disinterested is beyond our control.

The surgery or hospital is not the norm for patients. For staff it is your work place and you will hopefully be 'at home' there. In order to understand how a patient feels you need to remember what it was like when you entered the building for the first time, either for an interview or your first day of work. On a BBC Radio 4 programme about neonatal wards, a senior nurse talked about how she encourages nurses new to the ward to remember and retain how they feel and what they experience the first time when they walk onto the ward. She wanted them to realise that parents feel like that a lot of the time when visiting their tiny babies. She was attempting to get them to relate to their own feelings of strangeness, unfamiliarity and fear so that they would show empathy to parents who are seeing their premature baby hooked up to machines, in incubators and out of their reach.

It is essential that medical personnel recognise that patients often feel vulnerable about their need for care. Additionally, they can feel even more vulnerable because of the way that care is (sometimes) delivered.

Coping mechanisms

At this point it is worth offering you a chance to have to look at and to begin to understand how you cope in situations which are unfamiliar to you and where you do not have control, i.e. when you feel vulnerable. In this way you may begin to get a glimpse of and appreciate what patients experience. It may help you to realise where and when you feel comfortable in your work setting. Is it when your friends or trusted colleagues are around, when management support and trust your work, when senior colleagues behave with courtesy and kindness?

- When don't you feel comfortable?
- How do you find yourself treating patients when you feel uncomfortable, nervous or irritable?
- What coping mechanism do you employ to manage?

Ask yourself:

- How do I feel/behave when I need help or support from an unfamiliar person?
- How do I feel/behave when I am in an unfamiliar setting?
- How do I feel/behave when I am under stress?
- How do I feel/behave when I have to depend on another person?
- How do I feel/behave when I need something to be done?

The conclusions you arrive at if you answer these questions will give you a glimpse of some of the complexities patients experience during their interactions with medical personnel. By understanding our own vulnerabilities, we are better able to be empathic. Though we are often discouraged by societal norms to show our more vulnerable selves, being anxious, nervous or apprehensive is normal and nothing to be ashamed of. Having insight into how you cope in vulnerable situations can indicate to you the coping mechanisms you employ to manage challenging situations. Coping mechanisms serve a really important purpose. They enable us as individuals to walk out into the world every day, because they protect and enable us to manage daily encounters with other individuals, groups of people and the wider society.

You only need to think of the fight/flight response to recognise a well-understood coping mechanism. Walter Bradford Cannon, an American physiologist at Harvard Medical School in the 1920s, seems to have been the first person to give a name to the instinctive and physiological reaction in animals, including humans, that occurs in response to a perceived threat or attack – this he named the fight or flight response. The example often cited for the development of this response is that of early humans being under threat whilst surviving in a world full of dangerous creatures. The appropriate response to the threat of being eaten alive was either to stay and fight or to take flight. This response is both physiological and mental; the body under stress responds with an increased heart rate etc., and we need to use our minds to think our way through our reactions. When a person feels under physical or psychological threat today the fight/flight mechanism will still be an appropriate reaction. Sometimes it will be important to flee or actually physically fight but, in many circumstances, there will be a need to find the correct response to the situation that is evoking the fight/flight reaction. More recently it has been recognised that a further response to threat is that some people will not fight or flee, they will freeze.

It is important to understand that some of the ways we learn to cope are beneficial to ourselves and others; they enhance us. Other mechanisms begin as a means of protecting ourselves but ultimately may end up being harmful because their continued use impacts negatively on ourselves and others. For example, someone who has been bullied by a teacher may have made a conscious or unconscious decision to avoid anyone in authority or perceive those in authority as being bullies. The result of this may mean that they project their original negative feelings on to senior colleagues, thereby not relating to them as they are in the here and now. Alternatively, they may deny themselves the opportunity to progress for fear of becoming a bully themselves.

Projection is a means of deflecting unwanted feelings on to another person, when difficult feelings arise and threaten us in the external world. An example would be when an individual does not know how to handle their angry feelings, they accuse someone else of being hostile or having antagonistic thoughts.

Nearly everyone projects. It helps enormously to become aware of your own projections, both for your sake and for the sake of others. It is a challenge to be on the receiving end of a projection because you are not being treated as yourself, but rather someone has created their own picture of you and is treating you accordingly.

As a health professional you will be on the receiving end of projections. An individual's previous experience of doctors, midwives, nurses etc. will have an impact on how they view you and how they relate to you. You are likely to meet people who will perceive you as a threat because you have a degree of power, for example over what treatment they will receive, regardless of whether you think you are a threat. Projections can include positive feelings and attributes as well as negative ones, e.g. someone can endow you with being the expert, the one with all the knowledge.

An individual's projection may also be influenced by another person's perception. It may be that they or members of their family have had difficult dealings with doctors or nurses and they are going to guard themselves against what they expect to be negative contact with you. Some may assume they need to defend themselves from the outset and you may experience this as hostility. Others may 'give you the benefit of the doubt' but be cautious and wary of you, almost looking for you to start to be the inattentive, uncaring doctor they were expecting. Alternatively, they may have a positive image of a person in your role. They have had no reason to have any adverse attitude; it may be that they or their people have previously had positive experiences so even before they meet you, they will be either benign or expecting a positive reaction from you. For some people it will be their expectation that you are there for them and them alone. Others will be nervous of taking up your time and denying other patients time to see you.

Every individual you meet will have their own set of coping mechanisms, developed over time, with which they will defend themselves against perceived threats. Coping mechanisms have usually become integrated into what is defined as someone's personality and are not usually conscious ways of managing. A powerful coping mechanism is that of the critic. The critic begins to monitor how we behave, what we say and how we relate to others.

> Most of us have an internal critic. We may be aware of it or we may not. Our internal critic can have a powerful effect on the way with think about ourselves and consequently the way we live our lives. Sometimes our critic can be subtle and sometimes it can be demanding, sometimes it can be disguised as friendly advice or can be the motivator behind our act. We can deal with our internal critic in many ways however people tend to cope with it either by externalising their internal critic therefore becoming critical of others, or internalising it and becoming self-critical. (Both these ways of coping with the internal critic lead to ways of being which are not fully realised. In other words, we limit ourselves because criticising others

limits our relationship with them and criticising ourselves affects our relationship with ourselves).

(Hartley 2005)

The internalised critic can be so critical that in order to defend oneself against its negative voice another defence will materialise, i.e. the perfectionist. This additional defence of the perfectionist will have come about due to the experience of feelings of being unacceptable, being criticised and being wrong. These incidences of externalised rejection are internalised. A way of coping with life emerges that involves trying to ensure that the original experiences of rejection are never repeated.

If one can live within the perfectionist's standards, then one is safe from the feelings of being wrong and from powerful feelings of shame. Those identified with a perfectionist will do all within their power to ensure that they, themselves, do not make mistakes. The standards imposed by the perfectionist are often so high that it is inevitable that 'failure' happens. Failure can be something beyond an individual's control, e.g. they have an appointment, but transport delays make them late and being late is not within the perfectionist's frame of reference; therefore they are a failure and difficult feelings may arise.

It is understandable that doctors tend to be perfectionists. They will impose high standards upon themselves, not only because they do not want to make a mistake but also because the implications of doctors' mistakes can be profoundly serious. A big mistake might lead to someone's death and the possibility of being struck off the Medical Register and charged with manslaughter.

The 'perfectionist' coping mechanism is common and is particularly present in sensitive people who are often high achievers (or capable of being high achievers if they could get past their perfectionist!). The perfectionist has created a way of functioning where they try to ensure that they do not experience failure in any aspect of their lives. Feelings of failure can be triggered by anything that is beyond their control. They will have huge expectations of their ability to control life itself. If ever they do encounter failure, they will feel as if they are inadequate (which is what they fear). These feelings of inadequacies bring about feelings of shame and guilt.

It can be challenging for perfectionist women and/or their partners when they realise they do not have control over their fertility. If they do not conceive, despite them doing everything they can to get pregnant (they eat the right food, they don't drink alcohol, they use an ovulation kit), they will try harder and harder to do more of the 'right' thing. If the right thing is not successful, they will either blame themselves, blame each other or feel that their failure to get pregnant is a reflection of their inadequacy. On the other hand, women and their partners who are not identified with the perfectionist will be challenged by not getting pregnant, but they are unlikely to perceive themselves as being at fault.

As well as projections coming from personal experience, some will be derived from cultural expectations. We have met African patients who have said 'we expected this in Africa but we wanted better treatment in the UK'. They believed that a hospital in a high-income country would not provide an inadequate service, as compared with a low-income country.

It is crucial not to use an understanding of individual coping mechanisms and projections as a means of putting everything down to an individual. To paraphrase a quote from the novel *Catch-22* by Joseph Heller, 'just because you are suspicious it doesn't mean they aren't out to get you'.

It can be all too easy to blame individuals for societal and institutional biases. You need to have an awareness of the inequalities that exist in this society, and understand that it is not equal and classless. For example, poverty condemns people not only to being poor but often to being blamed for being poor. Being different despite laws against discrimination still means that those in any minority group suffer. Inequalities by their nature disempower people. As we have said earlier, the experience of being a patient is in itself disempowering, as patients do not often feel equal to the task of being in an environment where they are dependent on others for help.

Institutional inequalities have been highlighted in recent years. Institutional racism within the police force was highlighted in the aftermath of Stephen Lawrence's murder. Other tragedies such as the Grenfell Tower fire or the Hillsborough enquiry have shown that inequalities are inherent in our society. It is imperative that the health care providers consider what unconscious prejudices exist that contribute to patients (as well as staff) feeling disempowered.

It is not unusual for patients to report that they are amazed at their inability to speak in a medical setting. Many times, women have said something along these lines: 'I am a powerful woman in my work life but when I go in for a scan, I lose my voice'. This is not to do with her being shy: it is much more likely that she is intimidated by her surroundings, by a lack of any encouragement to form a mutually respectful relationship and perhaps by her fears about the results of any scan. Alternatively, other people are verbose, never really letting the sonographer speak or certainly not taking in what is said. This is another way of coping in an unfamiliar and therefore difficult situation, or it may be a defence against learning anything too painful. In each situation it is the responsibility of the health care worker to create a relationship of safety and equality.

As well as knowing yourself and your coping mechanisms in stressful situations, another way of gaining insight into what patients experience and how they feel is to read accounts of how individual doctors or other caregivers have changed their attitude because they themselves have been on the receiving end of medical care. Often, they will describe that they developed a deeper understanding of what it means to be a patient because of their own experience.

Insights into being a patient

Oliver Sacks was one such doctor. He was a physician, a professor of neurology and author. In his book *A leg to stand on* (Sacks 1984), he describes his thoughts, feelings and experiences of being dependent. Though his book was first published in 1984, it is still a good account of what feelings and vulnerabilities are encountered by 'becoming a patient' and many of his observations are still pertinent today.

Oliver Sacks was in his prime, pleased with his physical abilities and his prowess. He began a climb on a Norwegian mountain and as a result of attempting to avoid an encounter with a bull he fell and sustained a serious injury to his leg. He describes how challenging it is to go from someone who is at the height of his physical prowess and abilities one moment and then to lose that, becoming helpless the next. Instead of being full of vim and vigour in one moment, he was physically floored and he felt completely devastated the next. He portrays how this sudden change is challenging and difficult to understand. He finds himself trying to comprehend this and his mind tries to find reasons for this altered state.

This is relevant with regard to women who may be traumatised because they have needed to have emergency treatment during their labour and who cannot understand how they walked into hospital fit, well and 'only' in labour and then left weak, in pain and vulnerable. We look more closely at the impact of this phenomenon in the chapter on Intensive Care.

After imagining that he might die on the mountain because no one knew where he was, Sacks was rescued and was eventually flown to London and admitted to a hospital. Prior to his return to England he illustrates the impact on his morale and his ability to cope with how he was treated medically or how the Norwegian hospital staff related to him. His first encounter was with a nurse who was officious and a stickler for the rules who told him to stop complaining after he caused a fuss about being left with a rectal thermometer in place for over 20 minutes. He timed how long it was left in. Patients frequently take notice of how long they are left unattended.

Another encounter he has was with a doctor who he saw in his room as he emerged from sleep and the doctor was dancing around the room. He even leapt onto his bedside table, all in an attempt to reassure him that he would recover. The doctor showed him his own scars on his thigh to indicate that all would be well.

Dr Sacks describes how much the image of the young doctor stayed in his mind. He was unconventional and something about him represented the embodiment of wellbeing and strength. By being himself, he was able to impart such a degree of empathy that Oliver Sacks was moved. 'He didn't talk like a text book. His visit made me feel immeasurably better'.

He goes on to describe how upon arrival at a London hospital he coped with the surreal aspects of admission. He described how administrative and institutional expectations actually dehumanised him. Amongst the experiences he mentions are ones that left him feeling that he lost his individualism and that by being admitted as a patient he was robbed of his autonomy and he felt he lost his place in the world. He states that being in need of medical help made him feel as if he had forfeited his freedom because he needed to conform to the hospital regime.

However he quickly mentions that despite feeling this way, a nurse treated him with sympathy. This broke the feeling of being dehumanised by the system, and he felt like himself again. He illustrates just how transformative being treated as a person, an individual, rather than a routine patient, is. When this happens people can relax and feel like they are part of what is happening to them rather than being treated as an object.

It is over 30 years since *A leg to stand on* was first published. It is to be hoped that some aspects of care have changed and some better understanding of what it means to be a patient has developed, though clearly there is a lot of work to do before the Point of Care Foundation can become redundant. The changes that have taken place within hospitals do not mean that patients are any less scared about being admitted. Watching a relative leave you behind because they are not allowed beyond a certain point can be scary for some people; they are on their own in an environment that is alien to them.

Oliver Sacks writes that he looked at his chart towards the end of his hospital stay and what he read is that he had essentially an unremarkable recovery. You will need to read the book to fully appreciate how remarkable or eventful his recovery was, but what he says is that his recovery was full of events. Although the surgery he underwent was successful, he could make his leg function and had to wait for the trauma that his leg had suffered to begin to heal before he could apply any of his will to his movements. No one looking after him seemed to expect or understand this and as a consequence he suffered dreadfully without being able to speak to any medical person about this. This is despite him imagining that he would speak to the surgeon and rehearsed the conversation he would have with him, but it never happened because he was rebuffed when he attempted it.

Later he asked other patients who had similar operations or ailments if they had the same or similar sensations, or lack of them: most reported that they had. They never discussed it with the consultant who operated on them. Some felt rejected when they tried to do so, and some did not expect to mention it to anyone. This lack of insight by those looking after these patients, and the experiences of physical alienation produced by their injury and treatment, meant also that they (the patients) were left feeling isolated and potentially alienated because they thought there was something unique about their suffering. It simply was not recognised as a consequence of this type of injury.

Oliver Sacks discovered through his particular injury that the physical body behaves in a way which, until he was able to describe it, had not been recognised. As a result, a better understanding of the complexities of physiology and neuropsychology developed. These complexities can be included in the care plan following this type of surgery or procedure. They can be discussed with patients. They can be anticipated and an explanation can be given for the strange and alienating physical reactions.

This illustration of Dr Sacks' experience shows well what he felt like being a patient and also offered him insights into ways to 'humanise' and personalise treatments for patients with similar injuries to those he sustained.

In this digital age it is possible to have immediate access to how present-day caregivers learn from the experience of being on the receiving end of medical care. The Cleveland Clinic in America has produced a number of videos entitled 'Empathy Series', available on YouTube, that are designed to help further understanding of what being a patient means. The video, 'Patients – afraid and vulnerable, when caregivers become patients', shows medical personnel describing their feelings and responses to dramatic changes in their own health and what their experience was of being a patient (Cleveland Clinic USA 2013).

The video finishes with three statements which are paraphrased here. They reflect how those particular caregivers wish to use their own direct experience of vulnerability to provide person-centred ways of responding empathically.

- To have been treated with insensitivity can enable you to be more caring;
- Having faced one's own fear, it is easier to recognise it in others;
- Having been extremely ill and come back to life makes you realise how fragile life can be.

It is not necessary for all medical personnel to become recipients of care to provide person-centred care. But without staff feeling valued, supported and cared for, they can become insensitive or even hostile to patients who display characteristics they don't recognise as being legitimate. In order to address some of the issues that person–centred care brings to the fore, the Point of Care Foundation has introduced Schwartz Rounds, the origins of which are described on their website.

In 1994, a health attorney called Ken Schwartz was diagnosed with terminal lung cancer. During his treatment, he found that what mattered to him most as a patient were the simple acts of kindness from his caregivers, which he said made 'the unbearable bearable'. Before his death, he left a legacy for the establishment of the Schwartz Center in Boston, to help to foster compassion in healthcare.

I have learned that medicine is not merely about performing tests or surgeries, or administering drugs. . . . For as skilled and knowledgeable as my caregivers are, what matters most is that they have empathized with me in a way that gives me hope and makes me feel like a human being, not just an illness.

(www.theschwartzcenter.org)

From this experience, initially in Boston, Schwartz Rounds were set up to offer staff the opportunity to discuss the emotional and social aspects of working within healthcare. Schwartz Rounds take place in some NHS hospitals in Britain but they are as yet not a statutory requirement.

Oliver Sacks remarks 'how often had I myself, as a physician, mysteriously stilled the apprehensions of my patients – not through knowledge, or skill, or expertise, but simply by listening' (Sacks 1984). This simple yet profound statement illustrates that active listening is the first requirement: knowledge, skill and expertise can follow. It also implies that listening involves being fully present with a patient; listening to what is being said; what is not being said; having an enquiring mind and noticing how the person is presenting themselves to you. Listening itself is a challenging skill to acquire but which, once acquired, will be rewarding as it means relating human being to human being.

Creating a climate of inclusiveness within the NHS is demanding. It requires institutional change and individual responses to those on the receiving end of care. Staff have to feel important, considered and valued so that they can offer the best response to those who use their services. Satisfaction in giving and receiving care cannot be overestimated. The carer and the recipient can experience their true selves because they have recognised their mutual exchange as being valuable and valued.

References

Cleveland Clinic USA. Empathy series. 2013. https://health.clevelandclinic.org/empathy-exploring-human-connection-video/.

Cornwell J. We should see acute hospitals as places for healing. Chief Executive, The Point of Care Foundation. 10 May 2017.

Hartley M. 2005. leedspsychotherapy.co.uk.

Sacks O. A leg to stand on. Picador. 1984/1993.

www.theschwartzcenter.org.

3 Birth plans

This chapter discusses birth plans, what they may contain, and what may happen when a woman's experience does not match her plan. There are lots of debates and differing attitudes about the benefits or otherwise of birth plans. As we have highlighted throughout this book, issues of power and control are important in relation to pregnancy and birth. They are never more present than when it comes to delivery and the process of giving birth. It is at the heart of the debate as to whether birth is a natural process and therefore not requiring medical intervention. Lack of control and power are the two reasons quoted regarding the cause of traumatic births, i.e. unnecessary medical intervention and mistreatment by caregivers.

The Cambridge Dictionary Online (2020) describes control when used as a noun as 'the act of controlling something or someone, or the power to do this'. An alternative use of it as a noun is 'under control', e.g. everything is under control. When used as a verb the definition is 'to order, limit or rule something, or someone's actions or behaviour'.

Initially let's just look at the issue of getting (and staying) pregnant. For many centuries both men and women have used methods and contraptions to try to limit the chances of getting pregnant. However, it is only since the 1960s with the advent of the contraceptive pill that women have been perceived as potentially having the ability to 'order, limit or rule' their fertility. Having this control over if and when to get pregnant has had a huge impact for women who have been in societies where it is acceptable to limit the size of families.

In countries and societies where it is legal to terminate an unwanted pregnancy, this has also led people to feel that they can exert control. Despite this we want to acknowledge there are still many pregnancies that continue to full term where the woman will not have perceived herself as having control.

In circumstances where women have experienced control over their fertility, the act of 'trying' for a baby brings them into uncertain territory. Many women do not face the experience of uncertainty as they get pregnant within their own expected time frame. As a result, many will feel that they have had control over getting pregnant, as it happened when they *wanted* it to. There are women somewhat shocked to find that the first time they do not use contraception they become pregnant and this is not what they were expecting. These couples may feel that they had less control as it happened *before* they thought it would.

Other couples have to wait much longer to conceive and this can be a frustrating, difficult and worrying time for them. It is not unusual to hear women say 'all that time I tried not getting pregnant and now when I want to I can't'. This is a particular area that brings women, their partners and families right up against the issue of control as there is, certainly initially, nothing they can do but keep 'trying' and this is *not* what they wanted.

If a woman uses an ovulation kit and she gets pregnant, she will feel that she was in control via the ability to predict her most fertile time. However, there are many, many women who can testify that trying to get pregnant at your most fertile time of the month does not mean that you will conceive.

From these scenarios it becomes clear that control and what one wants are not the same thing. However, it is easy to feel as if they are one and the same, especially if you never experience anything that threatens this viewpoint. Equally, there are people who will never expect things to go well and who live in fear of things going wrong all the time.

Since it is clear that we humans are powerless to control conception it may also be true to say that it is not possible to control the birth of a baby. It is certainly possible to make plans regarding how you might like the experience of giving birth to be, but this does not guarantee that it will be that way. Pregnancy and giving birth are events that are full of risks. These include risks from the moment of conception – risks of an early miscarriage, a chromosomal abnormality, a late miscarriage or stillbirth. At the time of labour there are risks of complications. These risks are mostly beyond anyone's control and women are powerless to change the outcome. This does not mean to say that all steps that can be taken by caregivers to eliminate known risks should not be offered to women, but rather to acknowledge the risky business involved in creating and giving birth to a new human life.

We have discussed the fact that we all develop coping mechanisms to enable us to feel safe. It is understandable that pregnant women have conscious and unconscious coping mechanisms in relation to giving birth. Having a birth plan is an attempt to have some degree of control about the experience of being in labour and to have prepared in advance a way of coping with what is, for many women, a frightening experience.

Much is written about how obstetricians have taken over a biological process and some of the writings are quite vitriolic regarding the medicalisation of what is perceived as a natural event. Beverley Beech (2011) in her article for the Association for Improvements in the Maternity Services (AIMS) writes,

> Maternity care in the UK, as in much of the Western Hemisphere, is dominated by obstetricians, who have moved from a position where they were called in to assist with a problem labour to the current situation where they control the majority of pregnancies and births. They have done so by persuading the population that childbirth is inherently dangerous, that women's bodies do not function well, by undermining their confidence, by claiming that only obstetric care will guarantee a healthy baby and, worst of all, by carrying out what is now an international witch hunt to remove those midwives who practise real midwifery. As a result of this control, women's voices are often ignored.

There is a split between patients' organisations and individual patients' attitudes and that taken by medical personnel towards birth plans. Polarisation of this kind is an attempt to turn complex issues into simple matters; nature versus mechanisation. There is also a danger of creating an us and them culture with either side being seen as 'bad'.

One aspect of the debate is highlighted by Kelly Winder (2015):

> People are usually in one of two minds about writing a birth plan, or as some prefer to call it, their 'birth intentions' or 'birth preferences'. The two words, birth and plan, were always going to cause debate from the start. Who could possibly PLAN the way

their birth is going to unfold? Birth doesn't always go to 'plan', so some people think the whole exercise is a waste of time. I've even heard feedback from many midwives and obstetricians who think they are too. On the other hand, there are others who think having a 'Birth Plan', with that very name, is an important part of birthing women reclaiming power, giving them the right to have choice and the birth they hope for. They even feel that the words 'intentions' or 'preferences' are not strong enough words to convey that power and choice they believe all should have.

How a labour will progress is unknown during pregnancy when most birth plans are written. If a birth is uncomplicated, it can be called natural. If it is complicated, when there may well have been a need for obstetric intervention, it is not seen as natural, even though whatever it was that led to the intervention will probably have been very natural indeed.

Birth plans for many women have come to represent their ability to control or have their say in how they want the birth of their baby to be. For some, writing a birth plan is a device for trying to make sure that they do not have a traumatic birth. For others, writing a birth plan will be an attempt to ensure that they do not have a repeat of the traumatic birth they had before.

Depending on your viewpoint, the process of birth may be a natural event that will just happen or a potentially medical one that has to be organised and managed. For the majority of women, birth will just happen and whether or not there is a birth plan beforehand will not matter in the least. The contractions generally keep going, the cervix dilates and the baby descends through the pelvis whether the woman likes it or not.

The idea of making a plan for a physiological process may seem at first glance to be unnecessary since women who don't have a plan will still give birth. The baby does not stay inside the uterus because the mother hasn't made a plan for how he or she should come out. Equally, if the labour is obstructed and the woman requires a Caesarean section (CS), no amount of planning beforehand will make the baby smaller. If there is no alternative but to be delivered by CS, any planning then becomes medical rather than personal. The staff will know how to do a CS and will get on with it. They would not expect the mother to instruct them, any more than an orthopaedic surgeon would expect to be told by his or her patient how to fix a torn cartilage or a fractured hip.

So if, on the one hand, nature is in charge of the process and it will happen anyway, and on the other, nature fails (as nature is prone to do from time to time) and the midwives and doctors know what has to be done and how to do it, why make a birth plan? Are birth plans just wish lists or a waste of time, as referred to by Kelly Winder earlier?

In answering these questions we pose that a birth plan, from the patient's point of view, is not about whether the baby *will* be born, but perhaps more about how a mother would prefer to experience the process of her labour and giving birth; what can she do to influence the circumstances of her baby's birth; how can it be the best/easiest process; and what relationship she can have with those caring for her during labour.

Even if an orthopaedic surgeon does not need the patient to tell him or her how to perform the actual operation, we hope that the patient would have been involved in the decisions leading up to the procedure itself. It has been proven that patients' experience of the care they receive leading up to, during and after an operation has a huge impact on their recovery. Information and feeling involved in decisions about their health will influence their experience of care. Whilst patients are not asked to consider writing a plan for surgical or medical procedures there will nevertheless be a plan made at least by the surgeon and other related people and, if patients are not involved, it is not uncommon for them to feel excluded and that they will potentially suffer as a consequence.

Pregnancy and giving birth differs from other medical care. Childbearing is not an illness or an injury and so a different approach to patient involvement has evolved. The evolution of birth plans came about as an attempt to prevent women being disempowered in their experience of what is viewed as essentially a natural occurrence.

One of the first exponents of the birth plan was Dr Fernand Lamaze, a French obstetrician who in the 1950s popularised the idea of preparing for childbirth. The '6 steps' of Lamaze's teaching encourage women to learn about how to deal with pain and to feel confident about their ability to give birth without medical intervention. His six steps are simple and reasonable. They are:

1   Let labour start on its own
2   Move about during labour
3   Have someone with you during labour
4   Avoid unnecessary medical interventions
5   Don't lie on your back and follow your body's urges to push
6   Keep mother and baby together

These six steps would work very well in an uncomplicated labour. The potential dilemmas will arise if the labour is not straightforward, or if it doesn't start spontaneously by 42 weeks, or if some medical interventions become necessary.

Women's birth plans

By making a birth plan a woman is saying that she believes that she has some control over what is going to happen to her when she goes into labour. She believes that if she says that she wants something, or does not want another, then this is how it will be. Some of the points included in the birth plan may be straightforward, and easy for the staff to promise: 'I don't want to be looked after by students', for example. Others will be more arguable: 'I don't want to have an epidural' – it may be that that is the woman's position before labour starts, but when the contractions prove more painful than she has anticipated, should the staff continue to obey her original wishes or should they arrange an epidural if she then asks for one? Others will be much more difficult for the staff to guarantee: for example, 'I want a physiological third stage, without any drugs to make the uterus contract' when the woman says she has an objection to receiving blood and blood products.

Birth plans will usually be written during the pregnancy and will be discussed with a woman's midwife, obstetrician or both. This discussion will enable staff to have notice of any points in the birth plan that they feel are debatable or where they feel that the woman may not have been wholly informed about her options. Most of the time this discussion is straightforward because the birth plan contains nothing that is contentious or difficult to achieve.

Sometimes the birth plan will contain elements that the staff find a challenge, and then the discussion may take longer, or may take more than one meeting with the involvement of others. Staff are not being awkward when they find it a challenge – there will be challenging features in the birth plan that do not fit with their training or their Trust's policies. Take, for example, a case of a woman who had a CS for her first delivery and who wishes to have her next baby normally at home. Her midwife will be able to talk about how a woman with a previous CS is usually looked after when she is in labour, and how that would necessarily alter if she was at home rather than in hospital. The midwife would tell her line manager or supervisor to make sure that the woman was fully informed about the relative risks of this choice, and the senior midwife or supervisor would bring the case to the attention of senior midwifery and obstetric staff. Being forewarned about a planned vaginal birth after Caesarean (VBAC) at home means that staff on call can be prepared, as much as is possible, should the woman require urgent transfer into a hospital.

This example shows that through a process of negotiations, initially between the patient and her midwife or obstetrician, it is possible for a birth plan to be implemented. The plan has been inclusive; the woman and her caregivers have worked in unison; both sets of people are aware of the additional risks and are aware of what will happen if the birth is not straightforward. Problems are likely to arise when either the woman or staff feel excluded from the process.

If a woman's birth plan is fulfilled and her birth experience has included much of what was contained in her plan, then it is likely she will be pleased with the outcome. She may think that because she made the plan and it coincided with her experience that she is responsible for making it happen so successfully. If her labour and the birth of her baby do not go according to her birth plan she may be able to process the experience and feel that 'all's well that ends well'. She may feel like it was traumatic but not be traumatised by her experience.

For others, the fact that the birth plan 'failed', either because the mother did not insist on it being followed or because her plan was ignored, will feel like either she failed or others failed her. As a consequence she may well be traumatised. The difference in attitude will be proportional to her coping mechanisms and the support she is given by her caregivers.

Traumatic experiences in relation to birth plans are likely to occur for a number of reasons – we give some examples here:

- If a straightforward birth is anticipated and the patient has written a birth plan accordingly but something untoward happens, it can feel as if her plan is ignored. For example, if in labour it becomes evident that the baby is in an occipito-posterior position or 'back to back', and the labour takes longer and is more difficult, then women have reported that their plan was not implemented and no other explanation was given. Now it may be that it is the lack of information about what has changed or why the birth is protracted is as traumatising as the birth plan being ignored, or it may be both. This relates to communication by the midwife about what is going on during the labour.
- The reality of the birth differs so much from what was anticipated by the woman and the birth plan did not take this possibility into account.
- A woman's birth plan is so set in stone in her mind that any deviation means that something wrong must have happened, and this has a traumatising effect.
- Staff do not take any notice of what is written in the woman's notes, leaving her feeling ignored and helpless.

Birth plans, and their implications, can mean many different things for a patient:

- The notion of writing a birth plan = being in control of the situation
- Writing a birth plan means that an otherwise traumatic birth can be avoided

- If I don't have a birth plan then the birth may/will be traumatic
- My birth plan prevents trauma for me (but may cause trauma for the midwife who will be anxious about what may happen because of the plan)
- My birth plan may cause a different kind of trauma (i.e. obstetric trauma) for me
- My birth plan may cause trauma for my baby (for example if I am determined to avoid a CS)
- My birth plan may cause trauma for my children and my partner (i.e. if my uterus ruptures and I end up in Intensive Care, or worse)
- My birth plan deflects the staff from caring for other women because they are having to concentrate on me – how can staff talk about this without sounding bullying, or rude?
- My birth plan causes considerable anxiety amongst senior members of staff at the hospital
- If I stick to my guns about my birth plan then everything will be okay

Obstetricians' birth plans

There will be times when a birth plan has been written by an obstetrician in the light of a woman's previous experience, because the situation is potentially very serious and the woman wants the obstetrician to take control and remain in control. For example, if she had had her first baby by CS and then had wanted a normal delivery for her second baby, and she had suffered a uterine rupture during labour and her second baby had died, the plan for the third baby's delivery would be a CS before the due date by a senior consultant. Making a plan such as this is an attempt to ameliorate the woman's inevitable anxiety, and also to help the obstetrician believe that he or she has control in what is an obviously scary situation. Preparations will be made to try to ensure that everything goes smoothly on the day. The previous hospital notes will be requested and read, to determine exactly how damaged the uterus was with the rupture and how extensive the ensuing adhesions might be. Diaries will be consulted to work out which consultant will do the planned CS and which of his or her colleagues will be around that day to assist. Other cases might be discreetly rescheduled so that there is only one potentially difficult planned case that day. Meetings with a counsellor will be offered during the latter part of the pregnancy so that the woman and her partner can be helped with their fears, and there may be a visit to the labour ward to see the operating theatre and the recovery room beforehand so that they know a bit about what to expect. The on-call rota for a couple of weeks before the planned CS will be noted so that other members of the team can be alerted to the case; then, if the woman is admitted in labour, the on-call consultant knows whom to call for help if she needs to have her CS done as an emergency.

From a technical point of view there is a big difference between the birth plan made in this context and that made by a woman in her first pregnancy who would like as natural a labour as possible. One is filled with obstetric detail, including plans for the operation, cross-matching of blood, provisional booking of an HDU bed etc., and the other will stipulate choices about drug-free labour, possible positions for delivery and how the third stage should be managed. In essence though, both plans are doing the same thing: both involve people who care a great deal about what is going to happen making a plan in the hope that it will happen in the way that they have stated. Both parties feel that by making a plan they increase the likelihood of things happening the way they intend. The difference is that one is written from the perspective of knowing in detail what the risks are of not following the plan, and the other is written from the perspective of assuming that although risky events might happen, they hopefully will not.

People vary enormously in relation to their concept of risk. Most pregnant women will think about risk from the point of view of their own subjective experience, or that of people that they know, whereas health professionals usually tend to consider risk using objective evidence. (This may, of course, be against a background of individual professional experience – years ago I worked with a professor who refused to let anyone in his department use a Ventouse because of a disastrous delivery he witnessed during his training.) This means that any discussion about risk in the context of obstetric care can be tricky.

We will now go on to use as an example a birth plan for a VBAC as a defence against another traumatic birth, because this illustrates many of the points we would like to emphasise.

In some cases a woman who has already had a child will write a birth plan that is directly related to her previous experience of giving birth: a determined response to the last labour and delivery that says 'that is *not* going to happen to me again'. It may be the case that she had a birth plan for when her first baby was due, and her actual experience was not at all what she had stipulated. Her second birth plan is an attempt to claw back control over the process because her memories of what happened the first time are full of fear and disappointment. Take, for example, someone who had previously wanted to have a natural labour and delivery and who instead ended up with a syntocinon infusion, an epidural, a fetal monitor and a trial of instrumental delivery in theatre that failed and which was followed by an emergency CS at full dilatation. For some women, this experience will lead to a wish to have the next baby by a planned CS rather than risking having another emergency one. For others, it will make them even more determined than they were before to have the natural birth that they wanted in the first place.

Obstetricians are encouraged (by their hospital management, their clinical commissioning groups and the popular press) to try to reduce their hospital's CS rate. They will be under some pressure to convince women who have previously had a CS that they should have a normal delivery next time – a so-called vaginal birth after Caesarean or VBAC (something that used to be called a 'trial of scar' – a negative sounding term to say the least).

There are various factors that will influence whether or not a VBAC will be successful, and these should be taken into account during any antenatal discussion. They include the women's weight – VBACs become less likely with increasing maternal weight, with women who have a BMI greater than 30 kg/m^2 being 36% less likely to have a successful VBAC than those with a BMI under 30 kg/m^2 (Chandrasekaran et al 2016); her age – they are less successful in women over 40; whether she has already had a successful VBAC or not – as one would expect, if it has gone well once then it is likely to do so again (RCOG 2015); the dilatation she reached prior to her last CS – the VBAC is more likely to succeed if her cervix reached 9 cms; and if her cervix is already dilating on admission in labour – then she is more likely to go on to deliver normally, compared with if she arrives at hospital earlier in the process.

When discussing the pros and cons of a VBAC it is important to have knowledge of the circumstances of the first delivery: ideally one should have the hospital notes available in the clinic so that the details can be read. The previous surgeon may have written 'suitable for VBAC next time' in the operating notes, or conversely may have written 'not suitable for VBAC', for example because of an extension of the uterine scar into the broad ligament that might make future uterine rupture more likely. This detail may have been explained to the woman at the time of the previous delivery, but it is possible that either it wasn't explained well or that she doesn't remember the discussion, so having sight of the old notes is extremely helpful. Without them, there will be an assumption that a VBAC is to be expected when this might not in fact be the case.

To try to ensure that the VBAC process is as safe as possible, the obstetricians involved will hope that the following things happen: the labour will start spontaneously rather than being induced; intravenous access will be established once the contractions become regular, and a sample of blood is sent to the lab in case cross-matching is required; the use of syntocinon to augment the contractions will be avoided; the fetal heart will be continuously monitored once labour becomes established; vaginal examinations will be undertaken every four hours to ensure that progress is being made in terms of cervical dilatation and head descent; there will be early recourse to emergency CS if there is no progress, or if there are worries about the fetal heart pattern, or there is any suspicion that the uterine scar is about to open. The risk of so-called uterine rupture after one previous CS if labour starts spontaneously is only about 0.13–0.36% (RCOG 2015) but it is something so appalling that most experienced obstetricians will try hard to ensure it doesn't happen. This emphasis on safety makes for (in some eyes) a very medicalised version of childbirth, something that helps the obstetrician, and sometimes the woman as well, who may feel comforted by the medical attention to detail and the beep-beep-beep of the monitor. For other women all this is an intrusion on what should be a natural process, and the medicalisation of a VBAC brings back all that they felt was wrong with their labour the first time around, rather than it being a source of reassurance.

You may have a situation in a modern antenatal clinic, therefore, in which an obstetrician will try to encourage a woman to have a VBAC, but on the assumption that she will stick to the rules. The hospital will have a policy for how to manage a VBAC and the expectation will be that once the woman arrives on the labour ward contracting, the various steps described earlier will be followed. The obstetrician's 'birth plan' – the hospital policy – will be carried out in most cases: for other women, this proposed medicalisation of their childbirth will lead them to write a different birth plan altogether. They may accept some aspects of the policy but not others, or they may reject all of them, wanting to have the normal labour that they had wanted before.

Almost all of the medical trappings of a VBAC are put in place not to prevent a uterine rupture (this would be impossible – the only way to prevent a uterine rupture would be to do a CS before the woman goes into labour), but to alert the staff that a rupture is about to happen or is happening. This is why most obstetricians, especially those who have had prior experience of dealing with a uterine rupture and its aftermath, are so keen that the policy on managing a VBAC is followed. The avoidance of hormones is to prevent extra pressure being put on the uterine scar; the IV access is so that the woman can quickly be given fluid replacement and blood if she collapses; the fetal monitor is to alert staff to a rupture, since the fetal heart pattern will abruptly change when the scar starts to give way. Without the medical trappings one is jumping out of a plane without a reserve parachute – it may be okay in the end, but only in retrospect, and meanwhile it is terrifying. The woman who chooses a 'natural', unmedicalised VBAC of course does not see it this way at all – for her the medical trappings are an encumbrance to what should be a natural process and she believes that she will be much better off without them.

A woman who chooses not to follow the rules about a VBAC may be invited to a meeting at the hospital so that her plans can be discussed. Those at the meeting may include a senior midwife, perhaps an obstetrician, maybe someone from the hospital's risk office, and the woman herself. Her wishes will be discussed in detail and the statistical risks associated with her choices will be explained. The end result will usually be a written summary of the discussion – a so-called birth outside of guidelines – that can be given to the woman and circulated amongst the maternity unit staff to alert them about the woman's due date and the details of what she does and does not want.

Assuming that the woman is planning to have her VBAC in hospital, she will have been asked to come to the labour ward once labour starts. In a 'normal' VBAC she would be examined to see if labour had become established and if so she would have an IV cannula placed and foetal monitoring would be started. A midwife would be assigned to look after her who had no other women in her care so that the woman having the VBAC could have one-to-one care. In a 'natural' VBAC there would still be one-to-one care by a midwife but the other aspects of a 'normal' VBAC would be missing.

The midwife caring for the woman in labour will have been shown a copy of the birth plan and will know what the woman does and does not want. She will also know that the plan has been discussed (if not actually agreed) with one of her senior midwifery colleagues. Those senior midwives who met the woman beforehand and planned the 'natural VBAC' are not likely to be the ones that actually look after the woman in labour – the pressure is therefore on the midwife to work outside of hospital policy without direct support. Not only does she lack personal support in terms of the presence of a senior colleague, but also all the reassuring aspects of a 'normal' VBAC – the beep-beep-beep of the monitor, for example – will be absent.

The pressure on the midwife is even more apparent when a woman chooses to have a VBAC at home. The midwife is expected to behave with all her professional skill and accountability and yet is prevented from using the tools that would normally be there to help her do this. She is out of place – in the woman's home, not her work environment – and working in a manner that is not sanctioned by her hospital's policy.

She will hopefully have met the woman during the antenatal period and there will have been a discussion about the various points in her birth plan, so that the woman can be assured that the midwife understands her point of view and the midwife can be prepared for what to expect from the woman.

One of the main points to be discussed is the issue of transfer – in what circumstances would transfer from home to the maternity unit be advisable? In what circumstances would they be crucial? Ideally the terms for transfer would have been agreed beforehand between the senior midwifery manager and the woman, with the emphasis on prevention of a major complication rather than as a reaction to one that has already occurred. Indications for transfer should include the following: the presence of significant meconium in the liquor; a lack of progress in terms of cervical dilatation and head descent between one vaginal examination and the next four hours later; fresh, excessive vaginal bleeding; a persistent fetal tachycardia or bradycardia; a sudden cessation of uterine contractions; or alterations in the maternal observations suggestive of shock.

If there is failure to progress despite good contractions, transfer would be recommended since to persist at home in the light of a labour that is becoming obstructed would be to make uterine rupture and its attendant signs (sudden cessation of contractions, maternal shock) more likely. It would obviously be better to be in hospital if the uterus was about to rupture, rather than be transferred there once the rupture has already happened. The midwife will need to be able both to recognise that the labour is not going according to plan and also to convince the woman that this is the case and that transfer to hospital by ambulance is necessary without delay.

Community midwives all understand that they have a statutory obligation to care for a woman in labour regardless of how or where the woman chooses to deliver, and they accept their responsibility in an appropriately professional way, but there is no doubt that they are anxious about how the labour will go and what they might have to do. This is especially the case when the woman has decided to deliver at home more or less as a pro-test: after a discussion about the hospital policy on managing VBACs she has said, 'well, if I can't have my labour the way I want to have it, I'll have the baby at home instead'. Of course, the woman can make whatever choice she wishes and at home she can do what she likes, but it is her midwife who will bear the brunt of this decision and have to deal with its implications.

Partners and doulas

Women in labour will usually be accompanied, and their birth plans will have stipulated who is going to be with them. The birth partner will have a role to play as the conduit between the woman and the midwife. A birth plan may state clearly that information about, say, the progress of the labour, should be discussed with both the woman and her birth partner, and that decisions to be made about what is going to happen will be agreed between them both. This point may be clarified in the birth plan: 'my partner will con-firm that this is what I want if I am not in a position to be able to do so'. You can have a situation in which, for example, the woman will be asking for pain relief and her partner will be saying to the midwife 'no, she doesn't really mean that she wants pain relief, she says in her birth plan that she doesn't want any drugs'. The woman's birth partner acts as interpreter and protector: 'I know that she is saying that she wants an epidural but she doesn't really want one'. His role (in the example in which the birth partner is the baby's father) becomes that of 'defender of the birth plan'. This cannot be easy for him when his usual roles are 'lover of this woman' and 'father of this baby'.

The example given above demonstrates just how tricky it is to have a plan that has not been thought through, i.e. what happens if reality is different from the expectations that were included in the birth plan. How does the birth partner know to stick to the plan despite once experiencing actual labour, the mother is abandoning her or their plan? Who is the midwife to listen to? Is it the midwife or the doctor's role to suggest that the couple renegotiate the plan so agreement is reached? Is it likely that at this stage of the birth the mother is the one who is listened to and what the birth partner says is not heard, despite the fact that he may be adhering to the original plan? It is these kinds of circumstances that might lead a birth to become traumatic for the birth partner. Individu-als within a couple have felt abandoned by the other during labour, and they may harbour feelings against one another unless they are able to discuss what happened together.

Some women will employ a doula as a second source of support during labour. The Greek word *doula* means 'female servant', and doulas have been present during childbirth for centuries. A doula traditionally is someone, usually a woman, with no medical train-ing, but who would usually have had babies herself, who gives emotional support and encouragement to women in labour. Doulas first came to obstetric notice in the 1980s when research in Guatemala (Sosa et al 1980) showed that the presence of a doula in the labour room provided a number of beneficial effects for both mother and baby. The research was undertaken in a busy unit where it was normal practice for women to go through the first stage of labour unattended, to be helped by a midwife only when they started pushing in the second stage. The researchers found that women who had a doula with them during the labour had shorter labours and used less pain relief compared with women who did not have a doula.

At first this research was greeted with some scepticism amongst obstetricians, who believed that the doula effect was isolated to units like those in Guatemala where women were conditioned to go through labour alone and any help was better than nothing. This notion was countered when the research was replicated in a modern US hospital and the same beneficial effects were noted. Women who had a doula used less pain relief, were less likely to have CSs and their babies were less likely to have meconium aspiration and were able to breastfeed more easily than non-doula women. The study showed that a doula was helpful when she was supportive and kind as usual, but also that there was a beneficial effect to having a doula even if she just sat in the labour room doing nothing (Kennell et al 1991). It was felt that simply having someone else there changed the dynamic in the labour room so that the woman was able to labour more effectively.

Modern doulas are able to replicate this service, and are of great help to women who need extra support and encouragement in labour. This is especially the case with women who do not have a nominated birth partner and who otherwise would be labouring only with the midwife for support. Doulas are usually employed privately by the woman in advance of the due date and at the time of writing cost approximately £1,000.

One recent effect of the increase in the use of doulas in labour has been the phenomenon of the doula defending the woman and her birth plan against the midwives and (especially) obstetricians with even more vigour than the woman's birth partner. Birth plans nowadays may include clauses such as 'I will be accompanied in labour by my birth partner and my doula. All decisions about the management of my labour will be made by my partner and my doula, if I am not in a position to communicate. I do not want to have anyone in my room other than my birth partner, my doula and my midwife. I will not speak directly to any members of the medical team, who should discuss details of my labour and its management with my doula'. This takes the role of the doula to a new level. Where originally she was an untrained but sympathetic woman with personal experience of childbirth, she has recently become in some cases the gatekeeper to the labour room and the arbiter of obstetric decision-making.

This says a lot about some women's trust, or lack of it, in the hospital staff. They feel sufficiently anxious that their birth plan is followed and sufficiently uneasy about the likelihood of the midwives and doctors adhering to it that they employ another person to make sure that things go the way they want. This way of thinking also suggests that if doctors have direct access to women in labour then by definition it will not go according to plan – the involvement of obstetricians is seen as a *cause* of trouble rather than a *reaction* to it: the source of the problem rather than the means by which the problem is solved. It means that some women think that if they don't write a birth plan and that obstetricians are involved in the management of their labour, then terrible things will happen and their birth will be traumatic. The obstetricians' viewpoint is that terrible things happen in labour anyway and that they are best placed to sort them out. An obstetrician will seek to pre-empt problems rather than wait for them to arise, having had experience of what happens if nobody takes any pre-emptive steps – there will generally be more damage, more blood loss and more risk to the health and even life of both baby and mother.

The Nursing and Midwifery Council (NMC) has this to say on the subject of 'unqualified persons attending childbirth':

> The Nursing and Midwifery Order 2001, part 9 article 44 explains that it is illegal for an unqualified person to take the role of a qualified midwife. Article 45 further explains that no person other than a registered midwife or a registered medical practitioner shall attend a woman in childbirth (assume responsibility) unless in an emergency or in supported recognised training. An unqualified person is someone who gives midwifery or medical care but is unqualified to do so. This unqualified person may be an unqualified midwife, nurse, doula, partner, relative or friend who is not a registered midwife or registered medical practitioner. They may be present during childbirth but must not assume responsibility, assist or assume the role of the medical practitioner or registered midwife or give midwifery or medical care in childbirth. This is unlawful and may incur sanctions and a conviction.
>
> (www.mydoula.com 2012)

A traumatic birth is what the patient says it is.

I recall someone whose birth went according to her plan. Her healthy baby was born naturally in a midwifery-led birth centre, but then she ended up having a retained placenta. I was asked to see her some weeks after her baby had been born because she had had a 'traumatic birth'. I read the notes beforehand to become acquainted with the details of the case. The notes told the story of a normal labour and delivery, and then a retained placenta. All the usual things were done to try to encourage the placenta to come out (including rubbing up a contraction, getting her to empty her bladder, putting the baby to the breast, etc.) and when these didn't work the woman went to theatre for a manual removal. So far so normal, I thought. The woman's version of the story was anything but. She described the various actions used by the staff to try to remove the placenta as horrific, and she honestly thought that when the obstetrician examined her (to check whether the placenta was just held up in the vagina rather than stuck in the uterus) that she was going to die. When she was taken to theatre for the manual removal she believed that she would not survive the procedure and that she would never see her new baby or her partner again. Weeks later she was still haunted by the memories of all this.

She required a long debrief about what she had experienced and what had been done to her. In the discussion it was very important for her to ask me as the obstetrician whether she could have died. My response was 'you couldn't have died because you were in the right place, and the right things were done at the right time'. Having this confirmed had a profound effect on her. Nevertheless it was a long time before she could confront the possibility that she might be pregnant again in the future, because her equilibrium had been so disturbed by her experience of having a retained placenta. The impact of this case on me was to learn that what looks like 'normal obstetrics' to me looks like something else entirely to a frightened woman. Fear is what she says it is, and no amount of me trying to say that what happened to her was unfortunate but nothing out of the ordinary was going to make any difference.

What is the difference between women who have a difficult time during labour and delivery but who acknowledge that these things happen, and women who wrote a birth plan that went out the window? The first might be said to have had a traumatic birth and the second might not. Yet the first woman may not experience trauma and the second woman may well feel that she had a traumatic birth because her birth plan couldn't be followed.

Just as a traumatic birth is what an individual says it is, the impact of and ways of coping with the unexpected or unplanned aspects of giving birth are unique to each mother. It is hugely important to understand what it was that actually made a birth traumatic for whoever is traumatised, e.g. mother, father, or other birth partner or staff member. The example illustrated earlier indicates that it was not the fact that 'something went wrong' from the mother's point of view (as this was seen as an uncomplicated birth by the staff involved); it was that the realisation that her retained placenta, without appropriate care, could have caused her to die. This realisation of the potential fragility of life caused her, until she was reassured by an obstetric consultant in whom she had confidence, to lose temporary trust in many other aspects of her life. These included an inability to let anyone else look after her baby and to put unrealistic demands on herself as a first-time mother.

This case illustrates that all women come to labour with different backgrounds and perceptions, and all women will have markedly different reactions to what happens to them during labour and delivery. When we provide care during labour we must work according to our training and experience, but also bear in mind that what we do will be perceived very differently by different women. Giving care in some situations can be extremely challenging, but we must always do our best to be kind and sympathetic, remembering that what is a normal day's work to us is anything but to the woman in our care. If she says the birth was traumatic, then it was, whatever we may think.

References

Beech B. Challenging the medicalization of birth. *AIMS Journal* 2011; 23(2).

Cambridge Dictionary Online. 2020. https://dictionary.cambridge.org/.

Chandrasekaran S et al. Maternal body mass index has significant impacts on VBAC success. *American Journal of Obstetrics and Gynecology* 2016; 214: S239.

Kennell JI et al. Continuous emotional support during labor in a US hospital. A randomized controlled trial. *JAMA* 1 May 1991; 265(17): 2197–2201.

Mydoula.com. http://mydoula.co/wp-content/uploads/2012/08/NMC-Freebirth.pdf.

RCOG. Birth after previous caesarean birth. Green top guideline 45. October 2015. https://www.rcog.org.uk/globalassets/documents/guidelines/gtg_45.pdf.

Sosa R et al. The effect of a supportive companion on perinatal problems, length of labor, and mother-infant interaction. *The New England Journal of Medicine* 11 September 1980; 303(11): 597–600.

Winder K. www.bellybelly.com.au/birth/birth-plan-can-you-plan-birth update 5 December 2015.

4 Prolonged labour and shoulder dystocia

A prolonged labour would never feature as part of somebody's birth plan. Unfortunately some of the methods employed once labour is prolonged, such as the use of an oxytocin infusion, would not feature in a birth plan either. Obstetricians and midwives will be aware of this: they have to try to make the best of the situation once it arises. There are also features of a prolonged labour that in some cases serve as a warning about what might happen if the problem persists, and it is important that staff recognise those features and do something about them in as timely a fashion as possible.

For many women there will be a genuine fear that one intervention will lead to another (contractions hurting more than expected -> an epidural for pain relief -> the contractions slowing down -> an oxytocin infusion -> relative immobility because of all the drips and monitors -> even more delays in labour -> a trial of instrumental delivery which may or may not succeed). This fear is not an unreasonable one and it means that each intervention in a prolonged labour must be well considered and justified if it is to be acceptable.

It has been known for a long time that anxiety and prolonged labour are linked (Crandon 1979) and more recently a Norwegian study showed that women with a fear of childbirth are more likely to have a prolonged labour than those without a fear of childbirth (Adams et al 2012). Our aim should be to reduce a woman's anxiety during labour. Ideally she will have been able to express her anxieties beforehand with a trusted midwife or obstetrician. However anxiety about labour is understandable when some of our suggested 'treatments' will not have been part of her 'plan' and will only serve to make her anxiety worse.

Latent phase of labour

The latent phase of labour is defined by NICE (2017) as 'a period of time, not necessarily continuous, when there are painful contractions, and there is some cervical change, including effacement and dilatation up to 4 cms'. All maternity staff are aware that a normal latent phase can potentially last for days.

It can be galling for a woman to be told that she is 'not in labour' when she has been having painful contractions since the day before yesterday. When she tells the story of her labour to family and friends (and possibly to the obstetrician in the debrief clinic) she will say that she was 'in labour for days but they kept telling me that I wasn't'. NICE guidance recommends the use of individualised support and analgesia whilst also making it clear that the best place for women in the latent phase of labour is their own home. This should ideally have been discussed during the antenatal period, but it is likely that many women will have either not remembered what their midwife told them about it, or if they did, not appreciated how painful the latent phase contractions might be.

Delay in the first stage of labour

Delay in the first stage of labour can be due to cephalo-pelvic disproportion (CPD) or malposition. Both of these problems should be identifiable with clinical examination during labour, although increasingly obstetric staff are turning to the portable ultrasound machine to check the baby's position and to confirm that their diagnosis of malposition is correct. With a prolonged first stage when the baby is a normal size and in an occiput-anterior (OA) position, the delay may be labelled as a case of dysfunctional labour, especially if the contractions are infrequent or incoordinate. The word 'dysfunctional', although having been in common obstetric parlance for a very long time, does not lend itself to good communication with patients, with all its connotations of being 'flawed', 'not working properly' or 'not adequately dealing with something' and is best avoided.

There are natural methods for trying to deal with a prolonged first stage: encouraging the woman to be mobile and to try changing her position, doing your best to help her reduce her feelings of stress, and helping her in a positive and supportive fashion. If these methods do not improve the situation, an oxytocin infusion will be commenced. This aims to increase the strength and regularity of the contractions so that the baby is forced to flex its head and (hopefully) rotate and descend into the maternal pelvis.

There are potential pitfalls with oxytocin. It must be carefully titrated so that the contractions do not occur more than five times in 10 minutes, as too frequent contractions (tachysystole) will do more harm than good. It will often ramp up the pain so that the woman may want an epidural even before the infusion is started, and many will want one once it has begun to take effect. The anaesthetist may be busy with another patient, and so may take longer to arrive than the woman expected or wanted. This will only heighten her anxiety.

However much an anaesthetist may strive to make the epidural 'mobile', this will often mean that the woman is more confined to her bed than she would have wanted to be, and this relative lack of mobility will not help in terms of getting the baby to descend and rotate. An oxytocin infusion over a long period may also disturb the woman's electrolyte balance and it is important to keep an eye on her sodium level to check that she is not becoming hyponatraemic, which would be dangerous both for her and her baby.

You need to ask yourself before starting oxytocin, and certainly before allowing an oxytocin infusion to continue for more than eight hours, whether what you're planning is likely to work or whether it is too risky. Are you really thinking that a vaginal delivery is achievable and desirable in this case, when the physical signs might be telling you otherwise? For example, if the baby's head is persistently easily palpable above the pelvic brim despite many hours of contractions, or if there is haematuria because of the baby's impacted head pressing against the bladder, it is time to time to stop the oxytocin infusion and plan a CS.

Some women, even in the face of a lack of progress and signs of the baby's head becoming impacted, will want to carry on, in the hope that a couple more hours will make all the difference and result in a vaginal delivery. It is important to have as reasonable a discussion as you can about whether carrying on will be safe for the baby. In some ways, if the cardiotocograph (CTG) is already showing worrying signs, the conversation is more straightforward, at least for you: 'the problem is that the baby is already showing us that he's distressed and this will only get worse if we carry on'. If the CTG shows that the baby is coping well with the situation, the wisdom of a decision to call a halt now and do a CS is less clear. You might argue that in your experience, it is most unlikely that persisting with the oxytocin infusion for another two hours will result in a normal delivery, but the woman may well feel that she can be the one to buck the trend if only she is given the chance. Your task is to put your case clearly and accurately, with an emphasis on safety, both for the woman and her baby, and then (as long as the CTG is normal) wait a little while for them to make up their minds. While you're waiting you must document what you have said and the reaction you have received.

This is stressful for all concerned. From the woman's point of view, things are not going according to plan and she may feel that she needs to assert herself to try to change things for the better. It is however very difficult for her to assert herself when she is exhausted. From the point of view of the staff, there are other worries. Can we get this done before the end of the shift so we're not guilty of handing the problem on to our colleagues? Can we get this done quickly so that we can then get on with the delivery we need to do for the woman in the next room with the worrying CTG, or should we do the other woman's delivery first and risk this baby getting more impacted? Most importantly, can we get this done soon so that no harm comes to mother or baby? All this will be in your mind whilst you continue to try to make your case calmly, patiently and professionally. This is no small endeavour. It takes practice and (usually) a fair amount of experience to get this right, especially as you have to be able to be fairly flexible: whilst waiting another couple of hours may seem pointless but probably not dangerous in some cases, it will be genuinely very risky in others. You somehow have to get this across with the right use of language and the right emphasis on safety, without sounding paternalistic and bossy. It is of course something we can teach in 'skills drills' but it is also a good idea to take your junior trainee along with you when you are having these discussions, so that they can listen and learn.

Delay in the second stage of labour

Delay in the second stage may be a surprise, if the first stage has been normal with no concerns, or it might be the continuation of a prolonged first stage. If it was the latter, you should ask yourself whether you could or should you have predicted this. Of course these things are easy with the wisdom of hindsight, but there may well be plenty of clues that tell you that the second stage may not be straightforward. Those clues include a prolonged first stage, a persistently high head and the presence of haematuria.

There is a tendency to greet the announcement that the woman is finally 'fully' with a sense of celebration, but this may well be inappropriate. Just because the cervix is fully dilated, that does not necessarily mean that the baby is going to be delivered easily, and you must consider carefully how the labour has gone so far before committing yourself and the patient to an attempt at a vaginal delivery. You should consider the timeline of the labour, the partogram and what it tells you about the descent of the head, the fetal heart baseline and whether it has altered over these many hours, and the woman's remaining reserves of energy.

Remember that shoulder dystocia can be associated with a prolonged first and second stage of labour, as is instrumental delivery, so if you are embarking on a trial of forceps in theatre, be prepared for the possibility that the shoulders will be stuck. Any prolonged labour will also be a risk factor for uterine atony and postpartum haemorrhage, so be prepared for this, whether the woman has a vaginal delivery or a CS. At the very least she will require a syntocinon infusion and prophylactic misoprostol once she is delivered, and you should be ready to put in a Bakri balloon if necessary, either to prevent a haemorrhage or to deal with the one that ensues.

As with any proposed trial of instrumental delivery, you should ask yourself whether there is a realistic chance of the baby being delivered safely by forceps with minimal injury to the mother, or whether it would be safer in the long run to do a CS, bearing in mind the potential difficulties associated with a second stage CS. The thoughts going through your mind should be about *this* woman and *this* baby, not your ego or your unit's CS rates.

Shoulder dystocia

Shoulder dystocia is defined as a delivery in which additional manoeuvres are required to deliver the baby after the delivery of the head if gentle traction has failed. It is difficult to be certain about the incidence of the problem as it may be underreported, but it probably occurs in about 1 in every 200 births.

Whilst there are some known risk factors for shoulder dystocia, such as fetal macrosomia, many cases are not predicted and could not have been prevented. For this reason all maternity unit staff attend regular skills sessions to practise the necessary manoeuvres. That said, labour ward staff should be conscious of cases on their shift where the risk of shoulder dystocia is likely to be increased, so that they can be prepared. These include obese women, those who have been induced, and those with a long first or second stage or who require an instrumental delivery. For example, it would be good practice for the obstetric registrar not to leave the ward during the second stage of an obese woman known to have a baby with an estimated weight of 4.5kg and who has had a prolonged labour.

How to manage shoulder dystocia

Once the shoulder dystocia is recognised, the midwife will call for help and state clearly to the incoming team that this is a case of shoulder dystocia. Someone should take the role of scribe and document what happens and when. There are a series of simple measures that should be tried to resolve the problem (RCOG 2012): the legs are put into McRoberts' position, with one person on each leg; suprapubic (not fundal) pressure is applied to release the anterior shoulder; routine axial traction is used to deliver the baby. An episiotomy will not in itself release the anterior shoulder, but should be performed if necessary to allow the insertion of a hand for internal manouevres if simple measures are not successful.

Second line manoeuvres involve gaining access to the posterior part of the vagina, either to bring down the baby's posterior arm and deliver the posterior shoulder, or to press on the posterior shoulder to achieve internal rotation to bring the shoulders into the wider oblique diameter from where they can more easily be delivered. Some people find access to the posterior part of the vagina is easier if the woman is on all fours, and this is the best method if you had to deal with this situation at a home birth with hardly any or no help. In a hospital, with more people around, most would make the bed flat and take off the end of the bed once the woman's legs are in McRoberts' position to enable easier access. Obstetricians will tend to use the method they have found successful on previous occasions: for example, I have small hands, so finding the posterior arm and bringing it down is the method I favour.

Whatever method you choose, you should not keep trying to do it if it is not working, but rather start again and repeat what you have done before. Your aim should be to deliver the baby as soon as possible, without any excessive traction, and certainly within five minutes of the head having delivered.

Third line manouevres, such as cleidotomy, symphysiotomy and the Zavanelli manoeuvre, should only be attempted by very experienced practitioners with extreme caution, and in very rare circumstances.

What to do after a shoulder dystocia

A severe shoulder dystocia is probably the most terrifying of all the obstetric emergencies. This is especially true if you have little or no experience of it and you don't really know what to do. This is of course the case for the woman and her partner. One minute she is pushing as hard as she can knowing that she will see her baby very soon, and the next minute the room is full of people, her legs are being forced back up round her ears and there is a lot of pulling, pushing and (probably) shouting. A conversation afterwards with the senior obstetrician and neonatologist, once the dust has settled, is crucial, taking into account both her experience and that of her birth partner. There may have been time to warn them beforehand, especially if the baby was known to be large, but in most cases the shoulder dystocia happens out the of blue and this needs to be acknowledged and appreciated when you are talking to the couple.

A severe shoulder dystocia is also terrifying for the staff, and they need a debrief too. The most senior obstetrician involved in the case should gather the team together once the clinical work and paperwork have been completed, so that they can go through the details of what happened kindly and patiently. This is particularly important when some members of the team are inexperienced. An audit in our unit showed that whilst we were good at managing shoulder dystocia, and good at doing a debrief for parents, we weren't always very good at doing a debrief for staff.

Induction of labour

Women will require induction of labour for a number of reasons, including being significantly overdue or having particular medical conditions such as diabetes or obstetric cholestasis. When planning an induction you are essentially saying 'it is important that this baby is delivered sooner rather than later, and so if the induction process fails I will feel it is reasonable to do a CS to deliver the baby'. If you can't say that, you shouldn't really be planning the induction.

Very few women will specify in a birth plan that they want to be induced, and the process is at best unpleasant and at worst very upsetting, especially if it takes a long time. It might be prolonged if the cervix is unfavourable in the first place. If, for example, the baby's head is still 4/5 palpable and the cervix is long, posterior and closed, you should be questioning whether induction of labour is a good idea, as the process is highly likely to be either very prolonged or to fail altogether.

It is important to be honest with women about the potential outcome of induction of labour. It is not fair to tell them that they will be admitted to hospital on Thursday evening for induction and that their baby will be born on Friday. Whilst this might be so for some women, it will certainly not be true for the majority. In our unit a recent audit of induction of labour in primigravidae found that half of them ended up having a CS, either for failed induction, fetal distress or for failure to progress in labour. It is only fair to be honest with women about what might happen. Forewarned is forearmed, and so it is possible that being equipped with the knowledge that induction may lead to a CS means the mother will not have a traumatic birth experience, despite it being challenging.

Some women will request a CS if they reach the stage of otherwise having a post-dates induction. This will be either because of a previous bad experience of induction, or because of a fear of possible difficulties linked with induction, gleaned either from the experiences of friends and family members or from research. It is unreasonable and dishonest to suggest to women that induction of labour will always lead to a normal delivery, and it is only fair to talk through the possible outcomes in a frank and realistic manner. For example, a primigravida at 41 weeks with a non-engaged head who says she'd rather have a planned CS than an attempt at induction of labour is probably making a very good point, and after a careful discussion of all the pros, cons and options, it would be entirely reasonable to arrange a CS for her.

A debrief after prolonged labour

A debrief with an experienced member of staff ought to happen after a prolonged labour, even if the outcome was good, but definitely if the outcome was poor. For some women the consequences of a long labour, such as urinary incontinence, may not reveal themselves until later, and so knowing about what happened during the labour will at least help them make sense of the aftereffects.

When the woman is in a position to be able to listen and ask questions, you can go through what happened step by step, being prepared as always to stop and repeat yourself as necessary. The explanation should include details about the baby's position and the various tactics tried to help the labour along. When talking about this you should try not to imply that this was in some way the woman's fault: she may imagine that the baby's awkward position might be because she has an odd-shaped pelvis, for example. If she thinks that she is at fault it is kind to explain that this is not the case.

Sometimes the prolonged labour will have been at least partly as a result of the woman wanting to 'carry on for another couple of hours'. In such a case you have to be sensitive when talking about this, rather than apportioning blame or criticism. She has had a difficult enough time as it is, without you making it worse.

References

Adams SS et al. Fear of childbirth and duration of labour: A study of 2206 women with intended vaginal delivery. *British Journal of Obstetrics and Gynaecology* 2012; 1238–1246. DOI: 10.1111/j.1471-0528.2012.03433.x.

Crandon AJ. Maternal anxiety and obstetric complications. *Journal of Psychosomatic Research* 1979; 23(2): 109–111.

NICE. Intrapartum care for healthy women and babies. NICE Clinical Guidance (CG190) updated February 2017.

RCOG. Shoulder dystocia. Green-top Guideline 42. 2012. https://www.rcog.org.uk/globalassets/documents/guidelines/gtg_42.pdf.

5 Instrumental delivery

During an instrumental delivery the aim of the operator is to hasten the baby's birth whilst recreating what nature would do if nature was doing it properly. Fundamental to this is the ability to determine the position of the head and to work out how it needs to be altered to achieve the delivery, remembering the way a normal birth occurs: the baby's head is flexed in the occiput anterior (OA) position, descends through the pelvis and then after crowning the head is born by extension. So, if the head is not adequately flexed, the first part of the process must be to encourage it to flex. If the head is in the wrong position altogether, it must be encouraged into the correct position. If the head is still high in the pelvis, with some of it palpable above the pelvic brim, then it would be safer not to embark on an instrumental delivery in the first place.

There is pressure, either explicit or implicit, upon obstetric middle grade staff to try to reduce the rates of CS in their hospital, and as a consequence they may try to make sure that a woman delivers vaginally, using instruments if necessary. There will be circumstances when this will be a reasonable course of action and others when it would be best avoided, regardless of the CS rates. Experience can teach us when a vaginal delivery is unlikely to be safely achievable, because we learn to recognise when a labour is not progressing as it should, but this sense of when to stop (and when not to try an instrumental delivery at all) takes a long time to develop. Current training programmes do not lend themselves to the gradual development of obstetric intuition, which is why on-the-job, hands-on training and senior supervision are so important.

For some women the idea of an instrumental delivery is very frightening and something they would definitely wish to avoid. A birth plan may stipulate that they would rather have a CS than a forceps delivery. This may be because of her concerns about her pelvic floor, her baby's brain, or often both. She could harbour real fears about potential damage to her vagina, which would seriously affect her sex life and which may render her incontinent. Equally she may be very frightened about the possibility of the baby sustaining a skull fracture and damage to the brain, which would have serious life-long consequences. Whilst these outcomes are unusual, they are not out of the question. Any woman who seeks to avoid a forceps delivery in these circumstances should have her fears acknowledged, and should be told that a CS is a reasonable alternative. This approach will need to be seen in the context of the pressure upon obstetric units to reduce their CS rate. There will be an inevitable mismatch between the drive to reduce the number of CSs whilst at the same time treating each woman as an individual and in a manner that addresses her concerns.

Standard forceps

Standard non-rotational obstetric forceps come in pairs, with curved portions known as blades that go each side of the baby's head, and which are curved in the other direction to allow the passage of the forceps through the maternal pelvis. They thus have a cephalic curve and a pelvic curve. There are handles which lock together once the blades are correctly in place. If the handles do not lock then the blades have not been positioned properly. The appearance of a pair of forceps is alarming, since they look so big, and the name 'blade' suggests something sharp, when it isn't: both the sight and the name are best kept away from the woman and her partner as much as possible when you are getting ready for the delivery. It would be okay to say to the parents that you are going to help to deliver the baby with forceps, but try not frighten them by using the word 'blade' and try not to show them the actual forceps before you insert them.

The most commonly used standard forceps are Neville Barnes, Simpsons and Andersons forceps but there are hundreds of different types.

To carry out a forceps delivery correctly, the following must be in place:

F – **fully** dilated cervix
O – the operator must know the position of the **occiput**
R – **ruptured** membranes
C – **cephalic** presentation
E – deeply **engaged** head with none of it palpable above the pelvic brim; **empty** bladder
P – adequate **pain** relief

The doctor examines the woman's abdomen to make sure none of the baby's head is palpable above the pelvic brim. The woman is then put into the lithotomy position, her bladder emptied, and the baby's position defined by vaginal examination. Assuming an OA position, firstly the left blade is guided into place alongside the baby's head. Positioning the blade should be a fluid, graceful movement, without struggle or force. The trick is to hold the forceps handle parallel with the mother's thigh whilst placing the other hand in the vagina to protect the vaginal wall as the blade goes in. Once the blade is in place it should lie alongside the baby's head with the handle coming out at the introitus. The second blade is placed in the same way and the handles should then lock easily.

Once the blades are in place and locked the operator can begin delivering the baby, pulling at the same time as the women pushes with a contraction. It should be obvious with the first pull that the baby's head is starting to descend. Assuming this is the case with the first pull, the delivery of the head should be completed with a maximum of three pulls, i.e. during three consecutive contractions. If there is no movement at all after two pulls then you should give up.

The direction of the pull is important: not only outwards but downwards, because the shape of the maternal pelvis. This is helped by using Pajot's manouevre, where one hand holds the handles and pulls outwards while the other hand pushes the first hand and the handles directly downwards. In this way the direction of traction is at about 45 degrees to the horizontal until the head begins to crown, at which point the direction can come upwards. If an episiotomy is required it should be cut with the scissors between the blades at the height of a contraction as the head is crowning.

Ideally one should pull no harder than the force generated by one arm. Too much force would be very dangerous for the baby and damaging to the mother. It is tempting to try to brace yourself when doing a forceps delivery to be able to pull harder, but you must try hard to resist this urge. There should be no feet on the bed whilst you are pulling, and the woman's body shouldn't move down the bed.

A well-conducted forceps delivery should appear gentle and elegant, with the operator and the woman working together to help the baby come out. Sometimes, unfortunately, it is anything but: it is all too easy to struggle with locking the blades and then pull too long in the wrong direction. This is why it is so important that those learning to do instrumental deliveries are carefully supervised by senior colleagues until they are safe and competent. This means knowing when to stop (or not even start in the first place) as well as how and when to carry on.

Probably the most common reason for failure, or for a damaged mother and baby, is an inability to define the position of the occiput correctly. This is especially true if there is caput and moulding, making it difficult to feel the suture lines and fontanelles. If the baby's head is, say, occipito-transverse (OT), the handles won't fit and the blades won't lock unless they are forced to do so, which of course should not happen. If the baby is lying occipito-posterior (OP), the back of the head will be towards the back of the vagina and the face will be looking up towards the ceiling. If the position is mistaken for OA, which is possible if there is moulding and the fontanelles are not correctly defined, then the blades can be made to fit around the head, but when the head is delivered the large back part of the head will stretch the perineum much more than the face would have done. This can result in an increased risk of third and fourth degree tears.

It is bad practice to pull a baby out OP, unless the head is already well down in the mother's pelvis: it either means that you knew the baby's position but continued to pull it out that way anyway, or you misdiagnosed an OP position in the first place and assumed it was OA. You really shouldn't be doing a forceps delivery if you can't identify the position of the baby's head correctly.

Rotational forceps

The most commonly used rotational forceps are Kielland's forceps. These have a cephalic curve to accommodate the baby's head, but there is no angle between the blades and the handles so that they can be applied regardless of the baby's position (i.e. they have no pelvic curve). This means that they can be made to rotate within the mother's pelvis so that the baby's position can be corrected to OA and the head delivered in the usual way. The Norwegian obstetrician Christian Kielland invented them because trying to deliver an incompletely rotated head using conventional forceps was impossible (Baskett 1996).

Kielland's forceps have a sliding lock, rather than the fixed lock of the Neville Barnes, so that the blades can be placed if the head is asynclitic – in other words, if the fetal head has moulded so that one side of the head is a little further down the birth canal than the other. This will happen if the baby's head has been in an OT or OP position. One side of the lock has a small bump which should correspond with the position of the occiput. The blades are placed in such a way so that, say, the bump is at the back in the case of an OP position, and then, once the head has been rotated, the bump will be at the front, corresponding to an OA position.

The blades can be placed in the same way as standard forceps, though with an OT position one can use the technique of 'wandering' one blade over the baby's face, first inserting the blade posteriorly and then moving it over the face until it lies anteriorly. Once the blades are in position the head is rotated in between contractions. When the baby's head is OA, the delivery can be completed during the next contraction in the usual way.

Vacuum extraction

Vacuum extraction means a device (e.g. a Ventouse) is used to aid delivery of the baby's head by the application of a suction cup to the scalp. Because the suction cup is placed on the head rather than around it, the Ventouse does not add to the size of the head that is coming through the maternal pelvis and so in theory the risk of damage to the mother should be the same as with a normal delivery. Vacuum extraction is not used for babies before 36 weeks gestation.

A Kiwi is a smaller version of a Ventouse that can be used without any other equipment, to enable a baby to be pulled out more quickly. It should be used when the delivery needs to be expedited with the baby's head in a normal position. The cup of the Kiwi is placed on the flexion point of the baby's head as with a conventional Ventouse. The Kiwi is popular because it is simple to use and very portable.

Rotational Ventouse or Kiwi

A deflexed OP head can be encouraged to flex and rotate if the suction cup is placed on the baby's head at the flexion point, just anterior to the posterior fontanelle. Traction is applied downwards during a contraction, encouraging the baby's head to flex and rotate as it descends.

Manual rotation

To do this you need to have correctly identified the position of the baby's head as being OP or OT. Then (with adequate analgesia) you put your whole hand into the vagina so that you can hold the baby's head with your thumb on one parietal bone and your fingers on the other. Between contractions you should slightly disimpact the head and then rotate it to an OA position, using your other hand to steady the baby's body through the mother's abdomen as you do so. With the next contraction, the mother should push so that the baby is encouraged to descend and remain in the correct position.

Simulation training

Obstetric trainees can learn the principles of instrumental delivery, and practise the necessary manouevres, using specially designed simulators and mannequins (Sinha et al 2010) before they attempt the techniques in real life. This allows them to become fluent with the instruments and to learn how hard they can safely pull.

Trial of instrumental delivery

A trial of instrumental delivery (a rather unpleasant phrase) means that the obstetrician is not wholly confident that the baby can be delivered vaginally, and thinks that a CS may be necessary. In a situation like this it would be wrong to try to do an instrumental delivery in the labour room, fail to deliver the baby and then hurriedly move the mother to the operating theatre to do a CS. The correct thing to do would be to take the mother to the operating theatre, get set up as if a CS was going to happen, try to deliver the baby vaginally and then either succeed or move straight to the CS. If the baby comes out vaginally there is no loss of face and the obstetrician should not have been perceived as having taken the woman to the operating theatre unnecessarily. If a CS has to be done, everything and everyone (at least in terms of the staff) is prepared.

A trial of instrumental delivery would be chosen because the baby seemed to be particularly big, or in an awkward position, such as OP. This may have resulted in the labour becoming obstructed despite the cervix being fully dilated. Signs of obstruction may include haematuria and a lack of descent of the baby's head even though the mother is pushing well. If the baby cannot be delivered vaginally then a second stage CS will have to be carried out. This is potentially difficult and is described in more detail in the chapter on Caesarean sections.

When you go to theatre for a trial of instrumental delivery the theatre staff will often ask which instrument you would like. The correct answer is 'I don't know until I've examined the patient'. The baby's head may be lower than before; it may have rotated since the last examination; it may be more obvious once the spinal is working that a successful instrumental delivery is highly unlikely and you should be going straight to a CS.

An attempt at an instrumental delivery that turns out to be unsuccessful should not result in perineal damage. This is because an episiotomy should not be cut until the baby's head is practically crowning, and the perineum should have been protected from tearing by the obstetrician. However there have unfortunately been cases where the obstetrician has thought that a vaginal delivery was achievable and then either cut the episiotomy too early or pulled with the forceps in such a way that the perineum was torn, even though the head did not descend.

I have known of at least one case in which there was an attempt at a Kiwi delivery, which turned into an attempt at a forceps delivery which resulted in a third degree tear, which was unsuccessful and in turn resulted in a difficult second stage CS. This should not have happened: the person doing the delivery should either have foreseen the likelihood of failure and proceeded to a CS sooner, or been supervised more carefully by someone with more experience. The potential problems with instrumental deliveries, and especially trials of instrumental delivery, explain why there is an increasing likelihood of consultant presence on the labour ward.

Changing from one instrument to another

Generally speaking, it is not good practice to change from one instrument to another when doing an instrumental delivery. There will be times where it seems sensible – for example, if the cup comes off during a Kiwi delivery and the head is almost crowning, and the fetal heart rate has slowed down, one might use forceps to complete the delivery in a speedy manner. In another example, one might have used rotational forceps to turn the baby's head and then change to a Ventouse or Kiwi to complete the delivery.

Ideally you should continue as you started, and you should not switch from one instrument to another if it is obvious that the first is not going to work: this implies that you chose the wrong instrument or even the wrong type of delivery.

The RCOG (2011) recommendation is that changing from one instrument to another should be avoided if possible, as the practice is associated with a greater risk of damage to the baby than the use of a single instrument.

When to stop

An attempted instrumental delivery should be abandoned if there is no progressive descent of the baby's head despite adequate traction with correctly placed instruments over three contractions.

Risks of instrumental delivery

Examples of genuinely traumatic instrumental deliveries provide some of the most terrifying accounts of childbirth that it is possible to imagine. Rushed attempts at placing forceps blades, forcing them to lock when they shouldn't, and pulling too hard for too long can all cause serious damage to the baby and the mother.

Generally speaking, vacuum extraction is more likely than forceps to be associated with damage to the baby in the form of cephalhaematoma or retinal haemorrhage, but forceps are more likely than vacuum extraction to be associated with damage to the mother's vagina and perineum.

Why might an instrumental delivery be traumatic?

It is fair to say that some instrumental deliveries are perceived as having been traumatic by the woman and/or her birth partner although to the doctor conducting the delivery and the members of staff present it is a straightforward delivery with no trauma at all. An example of this would be a woman I saw in a clinic for a follow-up appointment in relation to her Kiwi delivery, one of the results of which was a third degree tear. The Kiwi was used because of concerns about the fetal heart during the second stage of labour, so that those attending felt that the delivery should be expedited. The woman described the process by saying that 'the baby was ripped from me' when the notes document a normal Kiwi delivery with no undue force. Of course the presence of the third degree tear suggests either that the baby's head was pulled out too quickly or the perineum was not adequately protected. Looking at the notes and listening to the woman I wondered with hindsight whether an instrumental delivery had been necessary, because the fetal heart abnormality was not severe and the woman had been pushing well and had made very good progress. This begs the question whether the baby would have suffered if there had been a few minutes delay before he was delivered and whether the woman would have avoided a third degree tear if she had had a normal delivery. As it was, the baby was fine and the tear had healed correctly, but the woman was left with the feeling that this was not how things should have been and that she had been needlessly damaged.

What we are talking about here is perception: the perception of the woman is that her baby was pulled out of her in an unnecessarily violent manner, which caused her to have a potentially serious complication, whereas the perception of the staff is that the baby was helped into the world using a straightforward process so that any possibility of hypoxic brain damage was prevented. Both versions of what happened are understandable and reasonable. As the people doing the listening afterwards, we must do our best to acknowledge this without making matters worse.

For another woman the account of her daughter's delivery was more worrying, although again the story as told by the woman and her partner was not reflected by the hospital documentation. A forceps delivery was required, again because of fetal heart rate abnormalities, and initially the delivery was conducted by a middle-grade obstetrician with supervision from the consultant. When the baby's head did not descend the consultant took over the delivery, and pulled much harder. A very strong operating department practitioner held the woman steady on the bed to prevent her whole body being pulled down and off the bed as the consultant pulled on the forceps. Eventually the baby was delivered, and after some quick initial resuscitation she recovered well. When she was a few months old, she started waking in the night screaming. Whilst any other parent would have attributed this to teething, her parents worried that it was to do with some form of brain damage linked to her delivery. The baby underwent a series of investigations, the results of which were all normal, but it was a very long time before the parents' fears could be allayed.

If a woman had imagined and hoped that she would deliver normally, and then did not do so, her perception of the event will be shaded by the contrast between what she wanted and what actually happened. She may feel disappointment, or that she has failed, or she may feel anger and resentment towards the staff.

Any perception of failure can be altered by the attitude of the staff at the time of the delivery and by the manner in which they communicate with the woman and her partner about what is happening and why. Too often an instrumental delivery is accompanied by a lot of shouting in the guise of encouragement, but if the delivery is conducted calmly and peacefully, with someone (hopefully the doctor doing the delivery) quietly explaining what is going to happen, it can be an easier process for all concerned. 'OK, when the next pain comes I want you to push like you did before, and I'm going to pull. It will feel different but don't be frightened, we'll all help you . . . that's wonderful, you're doing really well'.

Follow up

Any woman who has undergone a difficult instrumental delivery must be seen the next day, preferably by the person who did the delivery, but if not by someone of sufficient seniority, so that her physical condition can be assessed and her questions answered. Before going to see her the doctor should check on the condition of the baby, especially if the baby had to be admitted to the neonatal unit following the delivery, so that the conversation with the mother does not start off on the wrong foot – 'Where's the baby? Is he with dad? Oh, I see, I'm sorry, I didn't realise. . .'

As well as the standard observations of pulse, temperature, blood pressure, blood loss and urine output, there should be a check on the adequacy of her pain relief and a prescription for laxatives and stool softeners so that she does not have to strain when going to the toilet. There must be a check of her perineum to make sure that her stitches are correctly apposed and that there is no vulval haematoma. The doctor should explain what happened and why, and answer all her questions. There should be a discussion about the likely date of her discharge from hospital and arrangements made for her to have the relevant painkillers, laxatives etc. to take home.

If the delivery was anything other than straightforward (and it may be, as we have seen, that the woman's feelings about this will differ from those of the staff), then there must be a follow-up appointment in about six weeks' time to ensure that she has healed correctly and to give another opportunity for discussion when she is in a better frame of mind to listen and to ask questions. This appointment may be in a general gynaecology clinic or may be in a special perineal clinic or postnatal debrief clinic. The doctor seeing the woman for follow up must have the hospital notes available for the appointment so that he or she is aware of the details of the delivery and of any problems with the perineal repair or the condition of the baby.

Future deliveries

The general approach regarding deliveries in the future is that women should be encouraged to have another vaginal delivery unless they have had an anal sphincter injury, in which case they could choose to have an elective CS (RCOG 2011). From a straightforward physical point of view this is reasonable advice, but a number of women will have been upset and traumatised by their experience of an instrumental delivery and will not wish to risk repeating it. In these cases, a meeting with a consultant obstetrician fairly early in the next pregnancy should be arranged so that the choices can be discussed well before the due date, and if necessary a date for a CS can be agreed.

References

Baskett TF. *On the shoulders of giants: Eponyms and names in obstetrics and gynaecology.* London: RCOG Press, 1996.

RCOG. Operative vaginal delivery. Green-top guideline No. 26. 2011. https://www.rcog.org.uk/globalassets/documents/guidelines/gtg_26.pdf.

Sinha P et al. Instrumental delivery: How to meet the need for improvements in training. *The Obstetrician & Gynaecologist* 2010; 12: 265–271. https://obgyn.onlinelibrary.wiley.com/doi/pdf/10.1576/toag.12.4.265.27619.

6   Perineal, anal sphincter and bladder injury

Vaginal birth means that a baby is born via one of the most intimate parts of a woman's body. A woman's vagina is hidden and there are psychological and physical implications to this hiddenness.

Some women have looked at and explored their vaginal area but others have not done so. Of those who have not, many would be shocked at the idea of seeing this concealed part of themselves. A study by a gynaecological cancer charity, The Eve Appeal (2014), found that half of young British women did not understand the basic anatomy of their reproductive system. Out of 1,000 women surveyed, just half of those aged 26 to 35 could locate the vagina on a medical drawing of the female reproductive system. In contrast, the majority of women aged 66 to 75 were able to label their body parts on the diagrams. Less than a quarter of women aged 16 to 25 felt 'well informed' about gynaecological health issues, and one in five young women were unable to name a single correct symptom of any of the five gynaecological cancers, which affect the womb, cervix, ovaries, vagina and vulva. Nearly a third of women aged 16 to 35 said they had avoided going to the doctor with gynaecological issues due to embarrassment. The study also found that young women were uncomfortable with the word 'vagina': 40% of 16 to 25 year olds said they used names such as 'lady parts' or 'women's bits' instead. Just under a half of all the women surveyed said they would find it difficult to talk to their female friends about gynaecological health, and two-thirds struggled to talk to their sisters.

An internet search of 'women and their vaginas' results initially in several sites regarding women's reactions to seeing their vaginas for the first time and then an awful lot of porn. Objectification of women and their sexuality does nothing to encourage women to be interested in and to have positive attitudes towards their vaginas.

The fact that this often unexplored yet familiar area of the body can become hurt, damaged or altered during labour is challenging for many women. The wound caused by a perineal tear can be really painful, certainly initially, and the injury is in a very awkward place. It can be difficult to find a comfortable way of sitting, standing or walking until the wound heals.

If a woman does not know how her vagina looked prior to giving birth, the idea of looking at her 'damaged' anatomy can be horrifying. Even for a woman familiar with this area, the idea of looking at her altered vagina can be scary and can change her attitudes towards her body and her sexuality.

We will discuss the classification of perineal tears and their repair, and go on to expand on how women recover from them.

Classification of tears

Perineal tears are classified according to the nature and extent of the injury. These definitions are from the RCOG guideline (RCOG 2015):

First degree tear: injury to the perineal skin or vaginal mucosa;
Second degree tear: injury to the perineal muscles;
Third degree tear: injury to the perineum including the anal sphincter; these tears are further classified as follows:

3a: less than 50% of the external anal sphincter torn;
3b: more than 50% of the external anal sphincter torn;
3c: both external and internal anal sphincter torn;

Fourth degree tear: injury to the external and internal anal sphincters involving the anorectal mucosa.

Anal sphincter injuries (i.e. third and fourth degree tears) caused as a result of childbirth are called obstetric anal sphincter injuries or OASIS.

Buttonhole tear is a rather dainty term used to describe a tear of the rectovaginal septum, without necessarily involving the anal sphincter.

Risk factors for OASIS

There are two main risk factors for OASIS which we cannot influence. One is the size of the baby – vaginal delivery of large babies is associated with an increased incidence of perineal trauma and OASIS because it is commonly associated with episiotomy and instrumental deliveries. The second is the length of the woman's perineal body: if the distance between the back edge of the vagina and the front edge of the anus is less than 2.5 cm, then she is more likely to sustain an OASIS than a woman with a longer perineum (Deering et al 2004).

A iatrogenic risk factor for OASIS is the cutting of a midline episiotomy, or the incorrect cutting of an intended mediolateral episiotomy. It has been known for a long time that a midline episiotomy (favoured in the USA as it is more comfortable) increases the incidence of OASIS compared with the mediolateral episiotomy more commonly carried out in the UK (Coats et al 1980). It has also been shown that the majority of mediolateral episiotomies are not cut at the correct 60° angle (Andrews et al 2005) and are instead too acute, increasing the risk of OASIS.

OASIS is more common with instrumental vaginal delivery compared with normal delivery. If instrumental delivery is required, vacuum extraction is safer for the perineum than forceps (Eason et al 2000).

Evidence about possible prevention of OASIS

Antenatal perineal massage can reduce the incidence of perineal trauma in women having their first baby (Labrecque et al 1999), but perineal stretching during the second stage of labour has not been shown to help. Other useful measures to try to prevent perineal trauma are the application of a warm compress to the perineum during the second stage of labour, and allowing the baby's head to deliver in a controlled fashion (Kapoor et al 2015).

Routinely cutting an episiotomy in an attempt to reduce the risk of a serious tear is not helpful and should not be done. This was clearly shown in a review of six randomised controlled trials on routine versus restrictive episiotomy (Carrole & Belizan 2004).

We know that from Abdul Sultan's study (Sultan et al 1993) that 13% of women having their first baby by a normal vaginal delivery have anal incontinence or faecal urgency, and 35% of women having their first baby have anal sphincter defects afterwards detectable by endoanal ultrasound. Having an elective CS will protect against mechanical damage to the anal sphincter but will not prevent subsequent incontinence, which may develop as a result of a combination of other factors. These include body mass index, straining due to constipation and ageing.

Repair of perineal trauma

A first degree tear will often not require suturing as long as it is not actively bleeding and the skin edges are apposed.

A second degree tear or episiotomy should be repaired using rapid absorption polyglactin 910 (Vicryl rapide) which will be quickly absorbed compared with standard suture material. The patient should have adequate analgesia before the repair is started. The damaged area should be carefully inspected before starting the repair, with examination of both the vagina and rectum to check the extent of the tear. The tear is repaired using a continuous stitch, starting at the apex of the vaginal mucosal tear, continuing down to the fourchette, closing the perineal muscles and then repairing the skin from the end of the wound back up to the fourchette with a subcuticular stitch. Care must be taken to close any dead space in the muscle layer, and to ensure that the remnants of the hymen are correctly aligned.

At the end of the repair the vagina and rectum are reexamined and any swabs that may have been placed in the vagina are removed. Swabs, needles and instruments are counted and checked both by the person doing the repair and by a colleague to ensure nothing is missing or left inside the patient.

Repair of OASIS

It is vital that a damaged perineum is carefully inspected with a good light so that the extent of the damage is correctly noted. It is recognised that OASIS can occur even with a normal delivery, but it is a breach of duty to fail to recognise an OASIS and so fail to carry out an appropriate repair.

The patient must be carefully examined in the operating theatre with a good light, once she has had adequate analgesia (usually a spinal or epidural anaesthetic). The extent of the injury is determined and the repair is undertaken by an experienced trained practitioner, or by a doctor in training under strict supervision.

If there is a fourth degree tear, the anal mucosa is repaired with interrupted 3/0 Vicryl. The internal anal sphincter, if torn, is repaired with interrupted 3/0 PDS sutures. In the case of a 3c tear, the external sphincter can be repaired by overlapping the torn ends of the muscle and stitching them with 3/0 PDS, having first mobilised the torn ends. In 3a and 3b tears, the external sphincter is not completely torn and so the tears can be repaired in an end-to-end rather than overlapping fashion. Following this the vaginal mucosa, perineal muscle and skin can be repaired as previously described.

The repair of a buttonhole tear should involve a colorectal surgeon and may require the formation of a temporary stoma so that the rectum is bypassed whilst it is healing.

For a detailed discussion of the correct technique for OASIS repair the reader is referred to the standard textbook on the subject (Sultan et al 2009).

Women with female genital mutilation (FGM)

Women who have suffered different types of FGM will require examination before or during pregnancy to determine whether they have a type 3 FGM which would need to be opened to allow a vaginal delivery. The gold standard is to open the fused labia minora during pregnancy so that it has healed by the time the baby is due. In practice the major-ity of women affected by FGM will refuse this, so the fused labia have to be opened by the midwife during the second stage when the baby's head is crowning – a technique sometimes called an 'anterior episiotomy'. Midwives need to be aware of what to do so that the fused labia can be opened before the head gets too low.

Failure to open the fused labia in time means that the baby's head will be forced down-wards and backwards, so the woman will be at risk of sustaining a third or fourth degree tear unnecessarily.

After delivery, any bleeding points on the edges of the cut labia minora can be diather-mied or oversewn with tiny fine sutures, but the labia cannot be reclosed: this is illegal in the UK and women should have been made aware that this is the case during the antenatal discussion.

Post delivery management of OASIS

Following the repair, women with a third or fourth degree tear require a course of anti-biotics (usually cefuroxime and metronidazole), pain relief (without codeine, if possible, due to its side effect of constipation), bladder catheterisation for about 24 hours and stool softeners.

They need an explanation, both spoken and written, about what has happened and about what to expect immediately, in the first few days and during the first six weeks after the delivery. An appointment must be made to see a specialist in a perineal clinic in six weeks' time. Ideally the woman will leave hospital with the date of the appointment when she is discharged. As we have said, knowing what to expect and that 'someone' understands what might happen is immensely helpful.

Perineal clinic

Women attending a perineal clinic require a consultation with a specialist for a discussion and examination. The scarred perineum should be examined to check that healing is as expected and that tenderness has reduced.

The clinic should be staffed by a urogynaecologist and a specialist nurse or midwife, with associated colleagues including a specialist physiotherapist, a continence nurse, a colorectal nurse and a psychosexual counsellor (Sultan et al 2009).

All women attending a perineal clinic should have anorectal manometry and endo-sonography to determine the adequacy of sphincter healing and function.

The impact on women

Women use horrifying imagery when describing the damage done during childbirth. One woman, when talking to us about her vagina and vulva, said 'it's like a car crash down there'. A character in a popular radio drama described to her daughter-in-law that whilst giving birth she had been 'cut to ribbons'. Both images are graphic and powerful.

A woman who had a third degree tear described being horrified by the scar and feeling ugly. Another woman who had a bilateral episiotomy and subsequent tears described her vagina as a mess. She said she had 30 internal and 30 external stitches. Both women talked about the initial pain being very challenging. It was painful to sit and so finding a comfortable position for breastfeeding was awkward. Both women identified themselves as having had a traumatic birth and their experience of third and fourth degree tears contributed to their trauma.

Because of the extent of their tears they were both initially separated from their babies for longer than they expected to be. One of them was left in the post-operative recovery room on her own because theatre and ward staff failed to communicate with each other and her husband was left literally 'holding the baby'.

Both women stated that they were not treated well at their follow-up appointments. Their experience of pain and their struggle were dismissed. Having your reality dismissed by another person is deeply insulting; it will either lead to patients being angry and potentially abusive or it will just silence those who are already struggling to have their voices heard.

One of the women had frequent vaginal abscesses: when she sought an explanation about this she was given many courses of antibiotics and told that these things happen. It was not until six years after the birth of her daughter that she decided she would pay to see a consultant privately. She had always thought that some of the internal stitches were the cause of her abscesses. Her inkling that this was the case had previously been dismissed by her GP and she had the same response initially during the private consultation.

For her it was significant that the consultant she saw was also the NHS doctor she would have seen at the time of her confinement had he not been on holiday. Additionally her 'private' appointment took place in the NHS hospital on the same ward as patients who were not paying for treatment. This experience did not feel very private to her. The consultant agreed to investigate further and she had a procedure under anesthetic for this. Three undissolved stitches were indeed found and removed. She felt vindicated in her own mind but also angry that she had not been listened to. She never received an apology of any kind, but other than receiving a bill for the anaesthetic (which she did not pay and which was never followed up) she did not receive a bill from the consultant. She chose to take this as a form of admission of error.

The woman mentioned first went every month to a perineal tear clinic where she saw midwives.

> I told them that I was in considerable pain down there. I hurt when I was standing, walking, I couldn't put tampons in and certainly couldn't have sex. They told me that often this pain was all in the mind and I needed to get over it. They gave me some anaesthetic cream to use to numb myself before having sex and told me to have a glass of wine. My husband was horrified at the thought of numbing me so that he could penetrate me.

After 14 months she saw a consultant who specialised in tears, who said 'how come I haven't seen you in 14 months? You've been to every department in the hospital and nobody sent you to me?' The woman said that the consultant went on to say it was obvious I needed a repair operation and that she understood why I was in so much pain.

This patient also talked about how difficult it was when she attended a hospital appointment for biofeedback, which included a rectal probe. Her symptoms of faecal incontinence, faecal urgency and flatus embarrassed her and she became tearful when describing them to the consultant. She was told she had no need to cry, was asked what her problem was and felt dismissed. 'My trust in medical people had gone and their interpretation of me and what had happened to me didn't reflect how I was feeling at all. The action of allowing that probe up me was really difficult and felt invasive'.

Both women talked about sexual intercourse being out of the question for some considerable time following their tears. The woman who had repeated abscesses connects the ending of her marriage 10 years after the birth of her daughter partly to the fact that she and her husband had become sexually incompatible. He wanted sexual intercourse much more than she did. This was due to the ongoing problems with abscesses and pain. Additionally she could not contemplate another experience of being in labour and when she became pregnant again she wanted a termination. She was told by medical staff that no two births were the same, but she was not reassured by this information. At no point was she offered an appointment to discuss the possibility of a CS, and consequently she terminated her pregnancy.

We have used the experience of just two women who had significant tears to illustrate some of the issues that arise. There are many other stories that we have heard that are variants on these.

Just as 'no two births are the same', no two women are the same, so it is impossible to generalise about how women react to a perineal tear. What is clear from these two illustrations is that tears are a serious business for the women who experience them. There should be no judgements about how well a woman will 'cope' with her injuries.

There is a need for information about the implications of a third or fourth degree tear, which should be given as soon as possible. This information needs to be given by a sufficiently experienced midwife or doctor who can put aside enough time to really talk with a patient. Some of this information should include a description of the immediate consequences and the long term sequelae.

One of the women we discussed only saw a senior midwife three days after her delivery, and to her it seemed as if that only happened because she had mentioned to a doctor that she was incontinent and 'that poo was falling out of me and into the bed and onto the floor when I was walking to the toilet'. She only later understood that due to her injuries she had been given a laxative. No one had told her. If she had known she would have had an understanding about what was happening – that this was to be expected and not some failing on her part, or even that she was so damaged that 'poo' would continue 'to fall out of her'. One of the things she mentioned was that once she was at home she worried about leaving the house because she was frightened she would be incontinent. She would not eat before leaving the house to try to reduce the chances of involuntary defaecation.

Gaining control of our bladder and our bowel are amongst the first stages of childhood that we encounter. Loss of voluntary control of these organs affects people deeply. For most people, having control and even more so losing control is more private and personal than sexual intercourse or their 'private parts'. It is a deeply sensitive issue and women need opportunities initially to understand and if possible come to terms with the impact of childbirth on their bowel and bladder.

Bladder function after delivery

Loss of bladder control is not usually caused by tears, but rather by the muscles in the pelvic floor becoming weaker. This will be either as a result of pregnancy itself or because of labour. Urinary incontinence is very stressful with both a physical and a psychological impact. It is not unusual to meet women who know exactly where all the toilets are on their way to work. For some their problems with incontinence dominate their lives.

We have seen women whose lives are blighted by the loss of control of their bladder. One woman held herself very tensely because she felt that if she relaxed then her bladder would give way and she imagined it falling down through her vagina. The only way she felt she had control was never to relax.

Another woman felt her life was ruined because she had lost the ability to dance, run or laugh without leaking urine. She found it hard that this problem had been caused during the birth of her son. She was another woman who could not consider another pregnancy if the problem was to be exacerbated by another birth.

There is a real need for a women's health physiotherapist to be available for women who have bladder problems after childbirth, to advise on pelvic floor muscle training. After an initial assessment with a physiotherapist, an exercise programme can be designed for women to follow. They can also be helped enormously by the use of the pelvic floor muscle exercise Squeezy App.

Mode of delivery following an obstetric anal sphincter injury

At the time of writing there is no clear evidence about the best recommendation for mode of delivery following a third or fourth degree tear. The advice from the RCOG (2015) is not at all didactic, suggesting that it is best to leave the decision to the woman and her obstetrician. Ideally this conversation should take place after the delivery at which the tear was sustained. This gives the woman a chance to consider her options carefully and think about them before having to make up her mind. It may be that she will not feel confident about trying to be pregnant again until she is certain about how the next delivery will be managed. Certainly the conversation should take place no later than early in the next pregnancy, perhaps after the booking visit, so that the woman does not have to spend weeks worrying about how her next baby will be delivered.

As with any decision of this nature it is important to read the old notes if possible, to see what was written at the time by the person who did the original repair. There may be an explicit instruction to a future colleague that the woman should consider a CS the next time, or alternatively that she would be suitable for another vaginal delivery.

The choices for the next delivery, barring any stipulation from whoever did the previous repair, are as follows:

1   Encourage another vaginal delivery, with a promise to guard the perineum and if necessary cut an episiotomy to try to avoid another tear
2   Encourage another vaginal delivery, with a promise that the baby's head will be delivered very slowly, probably in a pool, with the woman 'blowing the baby out'
3   Offer a planned CS

Version 1 is very much the traditional approach, working on the principle that a vaginal delivery is preferable to a CS and that not guarding the perineum would risk another tear along the 'fault line' of the previous tear. In version 1 the surgical intervention of an episiotomy is seen by the person doing the delivery as preferable to another 'natural' tear. Whether an episiotomy can be seen in this light by the woman experiencing it is open for debate, and as we have already noted, the evidence in favour of a 'routine' episiotomy is lacking.

Version 2 requires a confident midwife who has the trust of the woman in her care. The woman must be able to listen to the midwife and do what she says, when she says it, in an atmosphere of supportive encouragement and calm professionalism. The woman has to believe that she is able to deliver her baby without serious injury to herself when in the past this has not been the case, and the midwife has to have the experience to know that this is achievable.

Version 3 seems a pragmatic approach: the troublesome area is avoided altogether and the delivery occurs in a calm, organised way. It does nothing for the unit's CS rates, and brings with it a whole list of other possible complications, not least the impact on the next pregnancy. If one chooses a planned CS for a second baby having sustained a third degree tear with the first, it would be logical to request planned CSs for babies 3, 4 and so on, with all that that implies in terms of surgical risks and duration of recovery.

The correct approach would be to discuss the pros and cons of these choices with the woman, so that she is able to make a decision which is right for her. Some will be able to make their minds up quickly about what they want to do, whereas others will find the decision more difficult. They may need more time, and more evidence, but what evidence there is on the subject may not always be helpful. It is important that a woman making her mind up about delivery has a named individual with whom she can discuss her options as much as she needs.

The ongoing nature of problems caused by vaginal tears or bladder incontinence are either a continuation of birth trauma or can be the cause of trauma for women who would otherwise have described their birth experience as being okay. For women who have already experienced a difficult birth, the aftermath of having vaginal, bowel or bladder problems means that the trauma is continued, especially if they are not given appropriate or adequate support. If there are no further consequences to a traumatic event we are more able to manage the distress caused, because it had a beginning and an end. If there is no foreseeable end to pain or humiliation, then the trauma goes on.

No one should be told their pain is insignificant or that they should be dealing with their trauma differently. As always, care should be person-centred, which means listening with kindness and where appropriate referring to experts, even if there is a risk of a 'wasted' referral. If it was established by a specialist that there was no further intervention needed, the patient could feel more content because she would know that she had been given the 'all clear' and the appointment would not have been wasted.

The women we have discussed described how they were not offered appointments with doctors who could immeasurably improve their symptoms for some considerable time and without some major effort on their part. They experienced physical pain and emotional torment for considerably longer than they needed to. These types of experiences make the aftermath of a traumatic birth even worse, and lead to patients having less trust overall in the medical profession.

References

Andrews V et al. Are mediolateral episiotomies really mediolateral? *British Journal of Obstetrics and Gynaecology* 2005; 112: 1156–1158.

Carrole G, Belizan J. *Episiotomy for vaginal birth (Cochrane review).* Chichester: John Wiley & Sons Ltd, The Cochrane Library, Issue 3, 2004.

Coats PM et al. A comparison between midline and mediolateral episiotomies. *British Journal of Obstetrics and Gynaecology* 1980; 87: 408–412.

Deering SH et al. Perineal body length and lacerations at delivery. *Journal of Reproductive Medicine* 2004; 49: 306–310.

Eason E et al. Preventing perineal trauma during childbirth: A systematic review. *Obstetrics & Gynecology* 2000; 95: 464–471.

Eve Appeal. Report of the 2014 review of research supported by the Eve Appeal. https://eveappeal.org.uk/wp-content/uploads/2016/06/The-Eve-Appeal-Research-Summary-2009-2014.pdf.

Kapoor DS et al. Obstetric anal sphincter injuries: Review of anatomical factors and modifiable second stage interventions. *International Urogynecology Journal* 2015; 12: 1725–1734.

Labrecque M et al. Randomized controlled trial of prevention of perineal trauma by perineal massage during pregnancy. *American Journal of Obstetrics and Gynecology* 1999; 180: 593–600.

RCOG. The management of third- and fourth-degree perineal tears. GTG 29. 2015. https://www.rcog.org.uk/globalassets/documents/guidelines/gtg-29.pdf.

Squeezy App. https://www.squeezyapp.com.

Sultan AH et al. Anal sphincter disruption during vaginal delivery. *The New England Journal of Medicine* 1993; 329: 1905–1911.

Sultan AH, Thakar R, Fenner DE. *Perineal and anal sphincter trauma.* London: Springer-Verlag, 2009.

7 Surgical considerations including haemorrhage and transfusion

This chapter deals with surgical challenges in obstetric patients. Many of these will be predictable, even if not preventable, whereas others take us all by surprise. We will discuss practical points about the surgery itself, the necessary conversations with the patients before and (especially) afterwards, and some of the medico-legal issues.

Caesarean section

In the UK about one-third of CSs are planned or elective, and two-thirds are emergencies. The latter are categorised according to their urgency:

Category 1: there is an immediate threat to the life of either the mother or the baby, e.g. in a case of cord prolapse.

Category 2: there is maternal or fetal compromise but this is not immediately life-threatening, e.g. in a case of an abnormal CTG with suspected chorioamnionitis.

Category 3: there is no maternal or fetal compromise but the baby needs to be delivered by CS, e.g. there is failure to progress in labour but no sign of obstruction and the CTG is normal.

It is vital that the obstetrician arranging an emergency CS communicates clearly with the anaesthetist and theatre staff about the urgency of the situation. For example, if you are going to do a Category 2 CS for suspected fetal compromise, you should explain what time you are aiming to deliver the baby, so that the anaesthetist knows whether he or she has time to top up an existing epidural or whether a (quicker) spinal would be preferable.

Difficult CS after previous surgery

Repeat CS, whether planned or emergency, is common, and may be complicated by adhesions regardless of the number of previous operations. Difficulties with adhesions can be very severe even after one previous CS, whilst in other patients, for example, a fifth CS may be relatively straightforward. Adhesions from previous surgery can make access to the uterus difficult, because safe entry into the abdomen is a challenge. Once inside the peritoneal cavity there may be adhesions from the bladder and bowel that make a normal lower segment incision more or less impossible. One either has to divide the adhesions (or ask another surgeon to help you do this) and enter the uterus in the usual way eventually, or open the uterus at a higher level than usual to avoid the adhesions, risking more bleeding as a result of having to cut through the thicker upper uterine segment.

CS after a previous myomectomy should be considered to be potentially complicated because of the likelihood of adhesions. If this is a planned case, more time than usual should be allocated for it, with the anaesthetist warned accordingly in case they want to do a combined spinal and epidural (CSE) rather than a single shot spinal. It would be wise to have a colorectal surgeon on standby in case help is needed to dissect portions of bowel from the lower uterine segment.

The combination of lower uterine fibroids and adhesions may make access to the lower segment difficult and make delivery of the baby's head problematic. A high head in these circumstances may need to be delivered with forceps. If this is not possible, you can find the baby's feet (remember that feet have heels, whereas hands do not) and deliver him as a breech using the reversed breech manouevre (Jeve et al 2016).

There is an overall increase in the risk of complications related to the number of previous CSs, although these risks are difficult to quantify. A chief concern is the possibility of placenta accreta: if the placenta is known to be anterior and low, the patient should have a fetal medicine unit scan, after the 20 week scan but ideally before the third trimester, to exclude placenta accreta. The relative risk of placenta accreta is 35 times higher in women who have had a previous CS compared with those who have not had a CS (To & Leung 1995). If the condition is diagnosed during the antenatal period, arrangements should be made for the patient to be delivered in a tertiary centre with a 24-hour interventional radiology service to enable uterine artery embolisation prior to surgery.

Emergency CS for obstructed labour

An emergency CS is more risky than a planned CS for a number of reasons. There is a greater risk of blood loss, infection, damage to other organs and trauma to the baby. The risks increase if the emergency CS has been preceded by labour that has become obstructed.

In an ideal world one would have predicted the possibility of obstructed labour and carried out the CS before it happened, but this policy would to some extent require second sight, and would most likely result in an increase in the overall CS rate that for some would be unacceptable. Having said that, there are signs that the labour is becoming obstructed that should be recognised by staff, so that the option for an earlier rather than later CS can be discussed. These signs include some or all the baby's head staying above the pelvic brim despite good contractions, and the presence of haematuria because of the baby's head pressing against the bladder.

Obstructed labour might be complicated by the formation of a Bandl's contraction ring, named after the Austrian obstetrician who first described it, in which the thick, muscular upper segment of the uterus contracts so much as to form a ring between it and the thinner lower segment, which becomes dilated. The ring will typically form at the level of the baby's neck, with the head below it. Opening the uterus above the ring will not allow delivery of the head, and opening it below it will not allow delivery of the rest of the baby: one has to cut across the ring to free the baby, so part of the uterine incision must cross the ring. Attempting to pull the baby up out of the pelvis when the ring is still intact will result in possible humeral fractures or a brachial plexus injury. Anyone starting a CS for obstructed labour should predict the possibility of a Bandl's ring and be prepared to deal with it correctly, rather than being surprised and confused by its presence.

Why a second stage obstructed labour CS is difficult

There are particular difficulties associated with a CS carried out in the second stage of labour. Obstructed labour will often be because of a fetal malposition, for example the baby's head remaining in a persistent occipito-posterior (OP) position, with the back of the baby's head at the back of the mother's pelvis rather than at the front. In this position the baby does not flex its head and as a result the head does not fit into the pelvis as it should. A CS in this situation should involve a larger uterine incision to allow room for the obstetrician to flex the baby's head and deliver it without further trauma. The incision also needs to be higher up the uterine wall than usual because of the risk of ending up in the vagina rather than the uterus if the incision is too low, with the resultant increased risk of bladder damage.

One common problem with this kind of CS is that the requirement for a larger uterine incision is underestimated, and so tears or extensions from the incision ensue as the baby is delivered. So-called angle extensions go laterally, out into the broad ligament, involving the uterine artery and vein, and other extensions can go downwards, behind the bladder and into the top of the vagina.

In some cases, even with a larger uterine incision, there is difficulty in delivering the fetal head. Obstetricians (if right-handed, and standing on the patient's right side) will typically try to release the fetal head first with the right hand, then with the left hand. If there is no success the table can be tipped so that the patient is head down, and the anaesthetist could administer GTN or terbutaline to relax the uterine smooth muscle, although the data suggest that these measures may not be better than a placebo, and will increase the likelihood of excessive bleeding (Morgan et al 2002). One should extend the uterine incision in a J-shape, find the baby's feet and do the reverse breech manoeuvre. Releasing the baby's body from the uterus in this way will immediately cause disimpaction of the head, which will then rise out of the pelvis easily.

A second stage CS will have to be carried out after a failed instrumental delivery. Until fairly recently it had been common practice for the obstetrician to push the baby's head back up the vagina after a failed instrumental delivery to facilitate delivery of the head at CS. Similarly, some obstetricians have asked someone else (usually a midwife) to push the baby's head up the vagina during a CS if they have been unable to disimpact it from the pelvis themselves. This practice is potentially very dangerous, as it can result in skull fracture and possible brain damage, and should be avoided.

A safer method is the use of a fetal pillow. This can be inserted following a failed forceps delivery to help elevate the baby's head in the vagina, making it easier to deliver via CS (Singh & Varma 2008). It is a gentler technique than manual pushing, and avoids the risk of skull fracture.

The patient will have been in labour for a long time and the uterus will be less able to contract effectively, so there will be an increased risk of blood loss because of uterine atony once the baby and placenta are delivered. This should be anticipated, and the patient given a bolus of oxytocin followed by an oxytocin infusion once the placenta is delivered. The patient may also benefit from rectal misoprostol at the end of the CS to help prevent atony. One cannot expect the uterus to carry on contracting effectively if it has spent hours trying to do so in the presence of an obstruction – it will need some help.

All of these problems are predictable if they occur in the context of obstructed labour. The obstetrician should clarify these possibilities during the team briefing before the CS starts, so that all members of the theatre team are prepared for what may need to be done.

Bladder, ureteric and bowel damage and their aftermath

The risk of bladder injury during CS is quoted at 0.08–0.9% (Tarney 2013). The RCOG consent guide to CS quotes a risk of bladder injury of 1 in 1,000, with ureteric injury being much more rare, occurring in approximately 1 in 10,000 cases (RCOG 2007). Bowel damage rates are difficult to quantify but will be more common in those who have had previous pelvic surgery (including a previous CS).

If there is doubt about a possible bladder injury at the time of a CS, methylene blue dye can be put into the bladder via the catheter to show up any leaks. A suspicion of bladder or ureteric injury must entail the involvement of a urological surgeon to come and assess the damage and carry out the repair.

Patients who have had a bladder injury repaired will require an in-dwelling catheter for at least 10 days post-op until a cystogram is carried out to check that the bladder has healed, and perhaps for much longer.

Ureteric injury may not be recognised at the time of the CS, and only become apparent when the patient presents with a pyrexia or flank pain. Treatment will require a stent and possibly a temporary nephrostomy while the repaired ureter heals.

Bowel damage recognised at CS requires the involvement of a colorectal surgeon to help with the repair, which may entail either a fairly straightforward resection and anastomosis or the creation of a temporary stoma whilst the injured bowel recovers.

Injuries to bladder, ureter or bowel will come as a surprise and a shock to the patient and her family, especially if they result in prolonged catheterisation or a stoma. A senior obstetrician must explain clearly what happened and what the patient should expect in terms of aftercare and potential complications. A follow-up appointment must be made, preferably with the same obstetrician, before the patient is discharged from hospital, so that her progress can be checked and her further questions answered.

Dealing with major obstetric haemorrhage

A major obstetric haemorrhage (MOH) is currently defined as the loss of 2,000 mls of blood or more during or immediately after delivery. A MOH call is put out when a woman has lost at least 2,000 mls of blood, or if she has lost 1,500 mls of blood and it is obvious that the bleeding is not immediately stopping. The MOH call is made to the hospital switchboard operator who then automatically triggers alerts to all relevant members of staff who will be able to attend immediately to help or, in the case of laboratory staff, get on with cross-matching blood.

MOH is most commonly related to uterine atony, and efforts to get the uterus to contract (rubbing up a contraction; giving uterotonics in the form of oxytocin, misoprostol and carboprost) will often be effective in stopping the bleeding without recourse to surgery. If the bleeding does not stop despite these measures, the patient will need to be transferred to the operating theatre for an examination under anaesthetic and possible open surgery.

A variety of techniques may be required and are described next.

Manual removal of retained placenta

If the reason for the MOH is that all or part of the placenta has been retained, the patient will need to be examined to see if the placenta is coming out through the cervix or held in the vagina. If it is not, she will require transfer to theatre for a manual removal, ideally under a spinal block.

If the placenta is not complete on examination, the uterine cavity must be searched to look for a retained stray cotyledon or succenturiate lobe.

Bimanual compression

If the uterus is atonic after the placenta has been delivered, the bleeding can be stopped by pressing hard on the uterus with both hands, one in the vagina and the other on the abdominal wall. One hand makes a fist inside the vagina and pushes up into the anterior fornix: the other hand pushes down from above to press the uterus forward towards the pubic symphysis. The inside and outside hands press firmly together to prevent further bleeding whilst the uterus contracts (Lindsay 2004). Sometimes bimanual compression will be all that is required to make the uterus contract and to stop the bleeding, but sometimes the uterus will remain atonic despite bimanual compression and further measures will be necessary.

Intrauterine balloon tamponade

This technique involves having a balloon filled with saline inside the uterine cavity, pressing against the uterine wall and preventing blood loss from the placental bed. It is inserted via the cervix with or without access to the abdominal cavity, depending on the circumstances. The balloon is filled with enough saline to compress the uterine wall and cause a tamponade: this may be up to 750 mls (Dabelea et al 2007). It is a simple technique (Mezei 2014) and will often result in cessation of bleeding from uterine atony without any further measures being required. The double lumen tube leading to and from the balloon means that the fluid can be inserted or removed whilst at the same time the blood coming from the uterine cavity can be measured. The balloon will usually stay in place for 24 hours, and then the saline will be gradually released until eventually the balloon is removed.

If the balloon is put in place during a CS, with a view to filling it once the uterus is repaired, there is a risk that the balloon's tubing will get caught up in the sutures used for the uterine wall repair, making it impossible to remove the balloon the next day without a return to theatre. It is safer to insert the balloon once the uterine repair has been completed.

Brace suture

The brace suture or B-Lynch suture is a surgical technique that stops haemorrhage from an atonic uterus by causing mechanical compression. It is essentially a stitch version of bimanual compression. It was originally described in 1997 after experience of five successful cases (B-Lynch 1997). Since then the suture has been used worldwide, with the advantages of being relatively simple to perform and allowing the woman to preserve her uterus for a possible future pregnancy. Many women have become pregnant following a brace suture and studies have shown them to have no adverse pregnancy outcomes (Cowan et al 2014).

Use of the B-Lynch suture in combination with intrauterine balloon tamponade also has been described (Diemert et al 2012).

Vessel ligation

There are a number of techniques for reducing uterine blood loss that involve blood vessel ligation. The simplest of these is uterine artery ligation, as one would do during a hysterectomy. The uterus will still be vascularised afterwards because of its blood supply from the ovarian arteries. The next step, if this was not successful, would be internal iliac artery ligation. Most obstetricians would enlist the help of a vascular surgeon if they were contemplating this measure.

Uterine artery embolisation

Uterine artery embolisation (UAE) can be undertaken as a planned pre-operative measure, for example if the patient was known to have a placenta accreta, or as an emergency procedure during a severe post-partum haemorrhage (PPH). UAE requires the expertise of an interventional radiologist and would not be available round the clock in most maternity units. Patients predicted during the antenatal period as being likely to need UAE (e.g. those diagnosed with placenta accreta) should have their care transferred to a unit with a 24-hour interventional radiology service.

Hysterectomy

If the bleeding continues to be severe, and if vascular ligation hasn't worked (or the bleeding is too rapid and excessive to make waiting for a vascular surgeon practicable), then the patient requires a hysterectomy. Most obstetricians in this situation would do a sub-total hysterectomy for speed, rather than a total hysterectomy, as the bleeding will usually settle once the uterine vessels are tied, and there would usually be minimal bleeding from the cervical stump.

Even when it is obvious that there is no alternative but to do a hysterectomy as a life-saving measure, the experience is profound and troubling. Our practice is to involve more than one consultant obstetrician when possible, for moral support as much as surgical assistance. However difficult it may be for us, this is nothing compared with the impact on the woman, who has to be helped to accept the fact that not only has her life changed out of all proportion with the loss of her uterus, but that without this operation she would probably have died.

Post-operative discussion

It is of course important to discuss what happened afterwards with the patient, once she is able to concentrate on what you are saying and ask questions. This conversation may have to be repeated, as it is not easy to take in complex details when worried and/or in pain. It is also good practice to arrange a separate 'debrief' appointment, perhaps six weeks or so after the delivery, when patients are better able to understand what happened and can ask their questions away from the anxiety surrounding the immediate aftermath of the operation.

The post-operative discussion of an emergency hysterectomy is particularly difficult, and will require more than one conversation, with the most senior person available. This is not a task to delegate to a junior member of staff, but you should consider taking your trainee with you when you are having this discussion so that they can watch and (hopefully) learn. There should be a step-by-step explanation of what happened and why, perhaps with drawings to illustrate what had to be done, what used to be there and what is now left behind. If, for example, the patient has had a sub-total hysterectomy, she needs to know that she still has a cervix and so will continue to need cervical screening.

Any complication of a CS, and any MOH, should be reported as a clinical incident. A serious incident will be investigated by the Trust and those involved will be asked to supply statements to aid this investigation. It is good practice to write a statement as soon as possible after a complication has occurred while you were on duty, while the details are still fresh in your mind. In that way you can supply a more or less contemporaneous account when asked by the risk manager to provide a statement.

Consent

Consent prior to surgery must of course include a discussion about the potential risks and what would be done either to reduce those risks or to deal with them should they arise. Many Trusts will use a standard CS consent form, such as that produced by the RCOG, which has figures for the various risks (RCOG 2007).

Ideally the person who is about to do the CS should obtain written consent, but if this is not possible, then the person obtaining consent should at least be someone who is capable of performing the procedure. The more complex the CS is likely to be, the more important it is that consent is obtained by the surgeon about to do the CS, or someone of appropriate seniority and experience.

The consent form allows patients to stipulate what they do not want to happen, and the surgeon can say what they will not do, as well as what they might have to do. This conversation will be different with different people, depending on the potential complexity of their case and their views on the surgical details.

Most patients accept that surgery is by its nature risky, and that complications may arise. What most patients will find very difficult is a complication occurring about which they had no prior warning. From a medico-legal standpoint, if you have warned a patient that there is a 1 in 1,000 chance of her bladder being injured during her CS, and then her bladder is injured and she needs a catheter for 10 days, she will be disappointed but will accept the situation. If her bladder was injured but she wasn't warned about it, and she finds herself needing a catheter for 10 days, she will be aggrieved and has every right to make a complaint and a legal claim on the basis of the surgeon's 'failure to warn'.

Obtaining consent in obstetrics may become more complex if the patient lacks capacity. This is almost certainly the case when a woman has been in labour for hours and has received mind-altering medication such as pethidine for pain relief. Even though it is difficult to discuss the proposed procedure in this situation, this does not mean you shouldn't try.

If a patient genuinely lacks capacity and the proposed procedure is urgent, you should use consent form 4, stating why the operation is in the patient's best interests and (if possible) including the signature of a colleague from whom you have sought a second opinion.

Pregnancy care in women who refuse a blood transfusion

Women should be asked at antenatal booking whether they would be prepared to accept a blood transfusion. Those who say no should be referred as soon as possible to an antenatal clinic to see an obstetrician so that this decision can be discussed and appropriate plans made. The purpose of this is not to try to talk her into accepting blood (a task that is sure to be unsuccessful), but instead to prepare her for labour and delivery in the safest way possible in the circumstances and to assure her that her wishes will be respected.

Whether or not she is iron deficient she should be prescribed iron supplements (e.g. ferrous sulphate tablets 200mg bd or ferrous fumarate syrup 20 mls bd) to maintain her haemoglobin level during the pregnancy. In this way the inevitable bleeding at delivery will hopefully not render her too anaemic.

Women whose refusal of blood is based on religious principles because they are Jehovah's Witnesses will be able to obtain an Advance Directive from their church detailing what they will and will not accept in terms of blood products and other healthcare options. Those who are not baptised in the Jehovah's Witness church will not be able to get an Advance Directive but can still be clear about what they will and will not accept. A copy of the Advance Directive or her personal stipulation should be filed in her main hospital notes and on any electronic patient record, and a copy kept in her pregnancy book. The Advance Directive assumes that all women will refuse whole blood, but allows women to be clear about whether they accept blood products and whether they accept cell-salvage.

The process of cell-salvage produces packed red cells, but not plasma or clotting factors, so its use in those who refuse blood products is limited if the amount of blood lost is excessive. The loss of a substantial amount of blood will lead to disseminated intravascular coagulation (DIC) which would usually be corrected by plasma, which is missing from the cell-salvaged blood. A patient receiving a large quantity of cell-salvaged blood without accompanying plasma is at risk of further haemorrhage as a result of DIC.

Women who refuse blood should have a clear and detailed antenatal discussion with their consultant about the circumstances in which there might be significant blood loss, with special reference to any particular risks in her case (e.g. previous PPH, or the presence of uterine fibroids). The main points of the discussion should be documented in the pregnancy book. The discussion should include the treatments that would be carried out to prevent excessive bleeding (e.g. active management of the third stage) and to treat it if it occurred. For details about treatment the team should refer to the Jehovah's Witness Liaison Committee guideline on the management of obstetric haemorrhage in those who refuse blood (Hospital Information Services for Jehovah's Witnesses), which is a succinct but comprehensive account of how to conserve blood in obstetric patients who refuse to have a blood transfusion.

Something that must be discussed during the antenatal period is that in the event of significant bleeding there would be a much earlier recourse to emergency hysterectomy than in women who would accept blood. This is because one does not have the luxury of time to try out less drastic measures when the haemorrhage is continuing and one cannot give any blood. When this is explained honestly and clearly, most Jehovah's Witnesses will understand this, believing that it would be better to survive without a uterus than to die, but that it would be better to die than to have a blood transfusion. This is particularly important for those who refuse blood products (including clotting factors) as well as whole blood.

This conversation should occur in the privacy of the antenatal clinic consulting room, without family members or church representatives present, and the relevant issues and plans must be documented.

References

B-Lynch C et al. The B-Lynch surgical technique for the control of massive postpartum haemorrhage: An alternative to hysterectomy? Five cases reported. *British Journal of Obstetrics and Gynaecology* 1997; 104(3): 372–375.

Cowan AD et al. Subsequent pregnancy outcome after B-lynch suture placement. *Obstetrics & Gynecology* 2014; 124(3): 558–561.

Dabelea V et al. Intrauterine balloon tamponade in the management of post partum hemorrhage. *American Journal of Perinatology* 2007; 24(6): 359–364.

Diemert A et al. The combination of intrauterine balloon tamponade and the B-Lynch procedure for the treatment of severe postpartum hemorrhage. *American Journal of Obstetrics and Gynecology* 2012; 206: 65.e 1–4.

Hospital Information Services for Jehovah's Witnesses. Care plan for women in labour refusing a blood transfusion. his.gb@jw.org.

Jeve YB et al. Comparison of techniques used to deliver a deeply impacted fetal head at full dilation: A systematic review and meta-analysis. *British Journal of Obstetrics and Gynaecology* 2016; 123: 337–345.

Lindsay P. Complications of the third stage of labour. In: Henderson C, Macdonald S (Eds.). *Mayes' midwifery: A textbook for midwives.* London: Baillière Tindall, 2004, 987–1002.

Mezei GC. 2014. http://emedicine.medscape.com/article/2047283-overview.

Morgan PJ et al. Nitroglycerin as a uterine relaxant: A systematic review. *Journal of Obstetrics and Gynaecology Canada* 2002; 24: 403–409.

RCOG. Consent advice No.7: Caesarean section. 2007. https://www.rcog.org.uk/globalassets/documents/guidelines/consent-advice/ca7-15072010.pdf.

Singh M, Varma R. Reducing complications associated with a deeply engaged head at caesarean section: A simple instrument. *The Obstetrician & Gynaecologist* 2008; 10: 38–41. DOI: 10.1576/toag.10.1.038.27376.

Tarney CM. Bladder injury during caesarean delivery. *Current Women's Health Reviews* 2013; 9(2): 70–76.

To WW, Leung WC. Placenta previa and previous cesarean section. *International Journal of Gynecology & Obstetrics* October 1995; 51(1): 25–31.

8 ICU and anaesthesia

Obstetric patients in the ICU

It is now well recognised that spending any time on an Intensive Care ward can have a psychological and physical impact on an individual. Other members of a new mother's family are likely to have their own feelings about their wife or daughter being so ill to require such intensive care and treatment. This is even more so when this occurs following what initially started out as a straightforward labour. It can be the equivalent of finding out that your relative has been in a car crash; it is so unexpected.

The idea of ever needing to be on the receiving end of treatment in an Intensive Care Unit (ICU) or a High Dependency Unit (HDU) following labour will be the furthest thought from most pregnant women's minds. Whilst not common, some women do find themselves waking up on a strange ward, in need of intensive care and nursing following delivery of their baby. It is now understood that this experience has a profound physical and psychological impact on a mother, her partner and possibly her wider family. It is highly likely that to become so ill as to require intensive care is going to be a shock. The last memory a woman may have is of being taken to the labour ward theatre for a CS. Consider her surprise and dismay to discover she is surrounded by all the paraphernalia of machines and other critically ill patients.

Newly delivered women will be transferred to ICUs for a variety of reasons. Probably the most common are a major obstetric haemorrhage or complex surgery, and thankfully most will recover. For those pregnant or newly delivered women who die having been cared for in an ICU, the majority will have pre-existing cardiac disease or will have developed a pulmonary embolism (MBRRACE 2019).

ICUs are particular places, unlike any other ward, and will only be known by people who work there or who have had cause to visit a relative there. Therefore not only will there be confusion as to why women find themselves there, they will not necessarily recognise where they are. They may be alone when they regain consciousness, but the first face they see is likely to be the ICU nurse taking care of them. Disconcertingly, the next sight they see may be of a very worried husband or partner, who in turn may be overwhelmed by the whole experience. It is highly unlikely that her baby will be with her. As well as any physical symptoms she experiences, it may be that she will have to deal with emotional shock. Perhaps she will have no memory of being transferred to the ward.

Shock is an appropriate response to something unexpected happening. It is her body and mind's attempt to deal with a sudden and unforeseen event. One of the ways stress manifests is that it feels impossible to trust that any of life is predictable. For example, people who have experienced emotional shock may well think something along these lines:

'If this can happen to me, which was beyond my control, how can I feel safe again and how can I be sure that those people I love are going to remain unharmed?' After such an experience, a husband or partner may need to be very clear about communicating their whereabouts and how long they might be away. Should those expectations be altered or exceeded, it will be really important to communicate that to the person who has had the shock. Without clear communication they will imagine that the worst has happened and this may cause extreme stress. It may take weeks or months before they can handle anything unexpected happening again. If at all possible, those caring for them need to anticipate this and take all steps to alleviate their stress.

Women who have been in an ICU are taken aback by how exhausted they are and surprised about how long this exhaustion lasts. This is true even if they are on the ICU for a relatively short time. As well as exhaustion they will have other physical reactions: they may be panicky, have headaches or find themselves feeling tense some of the time.

Shock can also make one doubt and almost not recognise oneself: you may behave differently to situations compared with before. An outgoing woman may find that she has no desire to be social or find herself wondering 'what's the point?' This can be extremely disconcerting, as it is not something she understands and she cannot just 'pull herself together' and behave the way others might like her to behave.

These experiences may happen whilst the woman is on the ICU or they may happen gradually and continue over the following days or weeks, long after she has left the hospital. It is essential that labour and postnatal ward staff and community midwives have an understanding of the implications caused by being an inpatient on ICU or HDU. Without staff knowing what happened, the mother and her significant others are likely to suffer even more. Being informed and reassured that her experience is normal and appropriate given what she has been through can possibly alleviate the enormous burden of blaming herself.

Trying to make sense of a difficult experience often includes blaming oneself; it can be helpful to listen to what individuals feel responsible for rather than just telling someone blithely that 'of course you didn't do anything'. This response, whilst probably being technically true, is highly likely to silence them. If you are able to listen to what they are worried about then you will gain an insight into what is causing her continuing stress.

As well as having to deal with some or all of this, the woman will have had to manage being separated from her baby. She may initially feel too ill to be very aware of this, but it is hugely distressing not to be able to be the mother she will have spent months imagining herself to be. Staff in the ICU and those looking after her baby need to be in close communication and make every effort to arrange for her to be reunited with her son or daughter as soon as she is able. It is all too easy for the 'out of sight, out of mind' mentality to affect staff in different places, and for different disciplines to fail to feel responsibility for ensuring mother and baby bonding. Enabling this may take a bit of ingenuity but is well worth the effort.

Understanding what happened is hugely important. It is vital that as soon as possible a senior practitioner goes to see the woman and her birth partner to discuss with them what happened that resulted in admission to an ICU or HDU. You must be prepared to be patient and go at their pace. You will need to hear what their experience was and not just report what happened from a medical perspective. It may be that this initial 'debrief' will take place over a number of visits and you may need to repeat what you have previously said, as people in shock cannot instantly take things in.

Transferring to another ward from the ICU or HDU is another challenge. Sometimes women are taken back to the labour ward, as there is more chance of one-to-one care than on a postnatal ward. Whilst this is true, it is again essential that staff on the ward know what it means to have been in Intensive Care. Without an understanding of that, women are likely to be expected to be ready to be well enough to care for their baby without any difficulty. If this is the expectation, it can just compound the mother's feeling of isolation and loneliness as she has been robbed of the first moments and days of her baby's life. Likewise, if the mother is taken to a postnatal ward, she may experience envy and feel separated from women who have had no problems. From the outside she may look no different from them but she will be feeling poles apart, as her experience has had serious health implications or might even been have been life-threatening. There is a profound difference between her and most of the other women on the ward.

As well as the mother being traumatised by dramatic events during birth, it is worth mentioning the stress experienced by birth partners. They are witnesses to what has happened. They may have been with the woman during a long and protracted labour and they will also have watched maternity staff do whatever was required once the emergency became apparent. Often when there is an obstetric emergency, staff forget to communicate clearly with the patient or her partner. If they are not included it can be make an already extremely frightening experience worse. Sometimes the urgency means that the woman has to have a general anaesthetic and partners are excluded from the operating theatre. Very often there will not be anyone available to stay with the woman's birth partner, so he or she will have to find a way to deal with their fears of what is happening alone. This can be a truly terrifying experience; without forethought it is highly likely that they will have nowhere in the hospital designated for them to be and they will be left to 'hang around', with only their fears and imagination to keep them company.

If no one is available to help them through their fears then it is paramount that once the surgery has been completed someone from the team is dispatched to find them to explain what has happened. This has to include a report on how both baby and mother are, where they are currently, what will happen next, what to expect for both of them and perhaps most importantly when they can all see each other.

Even if the birth partner is able to be in the theatre during a procedure it may well be that they find this situation very frightening. An emergency CS is an alien experience for patients and their partners: staff are likely to be busy and the demands on them might mean that they forget to include the couple in their communications. Medical terms will be used and, because there is likely to be a 'curtain' between the couple and the operation, what is overheard may not make sense and by definition be anxiety provoking.

If the mother has to go to ICU immediately, the birth partner will meet the baby before the mother is able to do so. This is a loss for both people in the relationship, and again will not be what either had been planning. The anticipated shared meeting of their baby in the immediate aftermath of labour does not happen. Not only that, the father or partner is thrust into the immediate role of being 'mum'. Unless the baby is ill and needs to be in the neonatal unit then the baby will be discharged to go home with the birth partner. Hopefully there is a family network who can assist in the task of caring for a newborn baby. Not only will this be unexpected, but the birth partner may be in shock; they will be worried about what has happened to their partner and will have continuing concerns about her health. Maternity and ICU staff need to understand the impact a traumatic birth has on partners and in any debrief, time should be given over to them in recognition of their mental health.

Another complex aspect of emergency intensive care being needed at the time of a birth, is where a woman not only gives birth but also loses her womb, as in the case of a major obstetric haemorrhage that cannot be controlled in any other way. The hysterectomy will have been the last resort in the context of an extreme and life-threatening emergency that means that intensive care will now be required. Hysterectomy and birth are not compatible in normal circumstances. However, if there is no alternative, the removal of her womb is the only way to save a mother's life. It is unlikely that she or her partner will be aware of this occurring at the time of the procedure (as she will be too ill or the circumstances mean that she is unconscious). Awaking on an ICU without your baby and then having to absorb the news that your womb was removed is very demanding. We know from our work with women who have gynaecological procedures that those who are prepared for their operations and who have come to terms with any implications recover both physically and psychologically better than those who agree to necessary procedures unwillingly. In the case of an emergency hysterectomy after labour there is no way a woman can be prepared for all of the implications. She may need counselling to reconcile herself to her new status. Wombs hold all sorts of symbolism and individual women will have different relationships to their wombs. Some women feel having a womb is what makes them a woman. Becoming an infertile woman at the same time as giving birth is taxing and she may have to find a new self-image.

For some women it will not be enough for her to be told that without having a hysterectomy she would have died; she could have bled to death. She may be able to grasp the truth of this but what we know and how we feel are not the same; one is a concept, the other involves understanding and emotional acceptance. She has to take on trust that the operation was necessary. If there was no time to build a relationship based on confidence in her carers in advance, then a trusting relationship has to be formed with her after the event. Ideally this should be with the senior surgeon, who goes at the pace of the woman, and who does not think 'why is she worried about losing her womb instead of being grateful that I saved her life?'

The mother may have to grieve the loss of her womb whilst at a time of having all of the demands of a new baby. Her grief about having to have a hysterectomy may be put on hold whilst she tends to her baby, but at some point she will need to process her new-found status. No assumptions should be made about her reaction to her loss. Even if she has one child or several children, it is not anybody else's place to tell her how she should feel. At no point should she be told she is lucky to have her child or children; if that is how she feels it is for her to say, not her carers.

Anaesthetic complications

For some women it will be the anaesthesia involved in giving birth, rather than the birth itself, that they will find traumatic, perhaps because of a difficult past experience or because of stories relayed by relatives and friends. Some women will be terrified about the thought of being 'put to sleep', others will be convinced that having an epidural will render them paralysed and some will be afraid that even if they have an anaesthetic, they will be awake and feel everything. Some may have been prepared for possible problems with regional anaesthesia, having discussed this during the antenatal period with an obstetric anaesthetist, but for others their anaesthetic complications will come as a surprise and a shock.

A patchy epidural block, giving pain relief in some parts of the body but not others, can be at best a disappointment and at worst a real worry, and may necessitate further attempts at siting the epidural which can in themselves be traumatic. A patchy block may be expected in women who have had previous spinal surgery, but in some cases there is no obvious explanation. The woman may have pinned her hopes on having an effective epidural and be very upset that it has 'let her down'. Others will have not ever wanted an epidural in the first place, and so then if it doesn't work properly they can become even more upset and angry about having to have it.

A dural tap is a recognised complication of epidural anaesthesia, occurring in about 1 in 100 cases. It will result in a severe headache (post-dural puncture headache or PDPH) that is usually managed initially with rest, oral fluids and simple analgesia. During this time the woman may need extra help when dealing with her baby because her headache will worsen when she moves around. If the headache is still severe two days later the anaesthetist may treat the dural tap using a blood patch, inserting about 20 mls of blood one space lower than the original epidural (OAA 2018).

Spinal anaesthesia for CS has become the norm, especially in elective cases, and once the woman has got accustomed to feeling her body being moved about but it not hurting, she can start to relax and look forward to the baby's arrival. The spinal can, like an epidural, sometimes result in a patchy block, which will mean either another attempt at siting the spinal, continuing with the patchy block with added intravenous analgesia, or, as a last resort, converting to a general anaesthetic (GA). Although converting to a GA will deal with the pain, the result is that the birth partner has to leave the operating theatre and subsequent bonding with the baby by the mother may be delayed whilst she recovers.

A GA in a heavily pregnant woman is a potentially risky undertaking. A combination of a pregnant uterus pushing up against the diaphragm and increasing the chances of vomiting, large breasts getting in the way of attempts at intubation and the general air of anxiety about the theatre all conspire to make the anaesthetist's job more difficult and the sense of fear in the woman increase. Ideally an anaesthetic consultant will deal with this situation, or will support an experienced registrar in doing so.

The scrub team, including the obstetricians, will have scrubbed prior to the induction of anaesthesia, and the patient will be prepped and draped before she goes to sleep, so that the baby is anaesthetised for as short a time as possible. Seeing the surgeons scrubbed and ready to go will terrify some women, and the anaesthetic team has the challenge of making gentle, reassuring noises to their patient while at the same time concentrating hard on doing everything right. It is vital that all other noise in the theatre is silenced: there should be no chattering, no clatter of instruments, no sounds of impending panic. The senior obstetrician's task is to make sure everyone remains silent and refrains from fiddling with the patient's abdomen whilst the anaesthetic team does their job. You can start talking and operating only when you hear the anaesthetist say 'cricoid off' to the ODP. You do not want the inevitably traumatic nature of the situation made worse by unnecessary noise and fuss, much of which the patient will, of course, remember afterwards.

A very small proportion of women who have a CS under GA, probably about 1 in 600, will have some awareness of what is happening during the operation (OAA 2011). Whilst this complication is rare, it is acknowledged as a cause of PTSD and is the subject of a large prospective study (Odor et al 2020). A small proportion of women affected will have long-term psychological sequelae and will require professional help to deal with these. Women in this category warrant careful follow-up, with a summary for use by the team should she require an anaesthetic in the future.

References

MBRRACE-UK. Saving lives, improving mothers' care. 2019. https://www.npeu.ox.ac.uk/downloads/files/mbrrace-uk/reports/MBRRACE-UK%20Maternal%20Report%202019%20-%20WEB%20VERSION.pdf.

OAA. Your anaesthetic for Caesarean section. 2011. www.oaaformothers.info.

OAA. Treatment of obstetric post-dural puncture headache. Obstetric Anaesthetists' Association Guidelines. 2018.

Odor P et al. Protocol for direct reporting of awareness in maternity patients (DREAMY): A prospective, multicentre cohort study of accidental awareness during general anaesthesia. *International Journal of Obstetric Anesthesia* 2020; 42: 47–56.

9 Mental health issues

Fear of childbirth has been linked in many studies with a fear of losing control, and women with a high need for control in their lives will characteristically be afraid of giving birth. The importance for many women of being 'in control' is discussed in the chapter on person-centred care. This is not to say that women who like to be in control of their lives, and who seek to be in control of their pregnancy and delivery in the same way, have mental health problems, but simply that the innate unpredictability of pregnancy and delivery can push their capacity for control to its limits, and often beyond.

A study from Liverpool (Slade 2019) examined this topic in detail, by interviewing women with a fear of childbirth during their third trimester. The paper describes 10 elements that featured in the interviews, all of which have their basis in a need for control and a fear of uncertainty. These 10 elements are:

- A fear of not being able to plan for the unpredictable
- A fear of harm to the baby
- A fear of not being able to cope with pain
- A fear of being harmed during labour
- A fear of being 'done to'
- A fear of lacking a voice in decision making
- A fear of being abandoned
- A fear about whether the body is able to give birth
- A fear of loss of control
- A fear of birth and not knowing why

Being aware of these fears and understanding how they may manifest gives midwives and obstetricians the opportunity to come up with plans to support these women in an appropriate manner.

To maternity staff the notion of women being afraid of being 'done to' is both understandable and slightly galling. We like to think that when we 'do' something to women it is for a good reason and that something good will result from whatever it is that we have 'done'. We have to try to think about what is happening from the woman's perspective, and behave accordingly. You might think you are doing the right thing by imagining how you would want to be treated yourself, or how you would want your daughter to be treated, but in fact you have to put those thoughts aside and do your best to understand how *this woman* wants to be treated. The only way this can be done is by creating a trusting relationship where women feel safe enough to disclose their fears and feel able to discuss their mode of delivery with you.

The impact of traumatic birth on women and their families can be profound, and can cause a number of wide-ranging symptoms and problems. These can include:

- A detachment from the baby, with a difficulty in bonding
- A change in the relationship between the woman and her partner, with a likelihood of reduced closeness including less sexual intimacy
- An anger with doctors and midwives, with a lack of trust in relation to any professional from the maternity services and perhaps health professionals in general
- Flashbacks about the trauma, with intrusive thoughts and nightmares
- The avoidance of anything that might trigger flashbacks to the original trauma, including medical procedures such as smear tests, television programmes about childbirth or pregnant friends
- The avoidance of a further pregnancy, for fear of the same thing happening again
- As a consequence, she may have only one child or there may be a long gap between one child and the next

The development of mental health issues affecting childbirth

Primary tokophobia (from the Greek *tokos*, meaning childbirth, and *phobos*, meaning fear) is fear of childbirth in someone who has never previously given birth. This is likely to be due to the woman having experienced rape or child sexual abuse: at least 63% of women who have suffered child sexual abuse will have a severe fear of giving birth (Wright 2019).

It is important to emphasise that women with primary tokophobia are *not* 'too posh to push'. Whilst there have been isolated incidences of women in the UK asking for a CS because they think it's fashionable (some years ago a woman walked into my antenatal clinic and told me that she wanted a CS because that was how Victoria Beckham had had her babies), they are very much in the minority. Women with genuine primary tokophobia are not making a lifestyle choice: more often than not they have experienced sexual abuse as a child, usually from a close relative or a family friend, and this has had an extremely serious and lasting effect. They are terrified at the thought of going through a normal birth and need to be cared for with kindness, understanding and professionalism.

Any discussion with women about their fears and their history risks causing a mental or psychological repeat of the original trauma, especially if the midwife or doctor frames their questions in an insensitive way or one in which the woman has to keep re-telling her story. It is unhelpful to think that because she is frightened of giving birth that there must be something wrong with her. Instead, we need to understand that something wrong has been done to her and the outcome has been long lasting and very serious. A helpful paper from 2017 describes the concept of 'Trauma-Informed Care', making the point that when talking to women who are frightened of childbirth we should not be asking them 'what's wrong with you?' but rather 'what happened to you?' (Sperlich et al 2017). By framing your enquiries in this way you are acknowledging that the woman's fears are as a result of what has been done to her rather than because of some inherent personal flaw.

I worked with a woman who was referred to me in her third trimester who not only was requesting a CS but she also wanted to be unconscious during the operation. The woman expressed how frightened she was of giving birth, hence her request for a CS, and she stated she could not imagine anything worse that being awake during it. As a counsellor in this situation and given the lateness of the referral there was no time to explore the possible causes for her deep fear. She did not perceive herself as having a fear, more it was that she could not stand the idea of labour or being awake during a CS. To have attempted to delve deeper with someone who was unwilling or unable to discuss the reasons for her fear would have gone against the person-centred orientation I adopted. Rather I worked with a consultant obstetrician colleague who explained the risks and complications involved in the procedure and the anaesthetic. Despite these concerns being made clear, the mother-to-be could not envisage any other form of giving birth. Consequently her CS was planned and executed according to her wishes. By working together with her, she was able to have the best birth experience possible for her. It was, for her, a great achievement.

Antenatal care for women frightened of giving birth should be provided by a small number of people – ideally one specialist midwife and one senior obstetrician. By arranging care in this way you can remove the risk of the woman having to keep repeating herself: each consultation can just carry on where the last one left off.

Plans for the delivery should happen fairly early on – certainly as soon as possible after the anomaly scan – so that the woman does not have to worry for weeks about what the arrangements might be. She may well want to have a planned CS. The updated guidance from NICE (2020) makes it clear that women with a fear of childbirth should be provided with appropriate perinatal mental health support during pregnancy, and if vaginal birth is not an acceptable option for them, a planned CS should be arranged. Maternity staff should not make life more difficult for these women by making them feel as if they have to jump through several hoops to qualify for a CS. As the NICE guidance states, if a consultant obstetrician feels unhappy about organising the CS themselves then they should ask one of their colleagues to do so instead. In units with a perinatal health multi-disciplinary team (MDT), a senior specialist midwife can make these arrangements.

During the third trimester you should discuss in detail the plans for the day of delivery, including what exactly will happen and who will be there. Ideally the woman's named midwife will accompany her from the time that she arrives at the hospital, during the CS itself and in the immediate postpartum period.

Remember that a planned CS is not devoid of reminders about past abuse. You need to think carefully about the details and consider what you can do to minimise the distress that these may cause. Take for example urinary catheterisation: this is usually done after the spinal has been put in but with the woman wide awake, with no screen, and with an assortment of theatre staff bustling about getting things ready for the surgery. This needs to be discussed with the woman and if necessary the technique can be altered so that, say, the catheter doesn't go in until the spinal block has been checked to be fully effective and a screen is put in place so the woman doesn't need to see what's going on. This arrangement may suit her best: alternatively she may hate the idea of something being 'done' to her that she cannot see and cannot prevent. You have to listen to her, talk to her and find out what she would prefer, without making any assumptions. In the same way, you should talk about whether she wants skin-to-skin contact with her baby during the CS – this might be something that she is really looking forward to, or something she would find very difficult. Again, don't assume that you know what she'll want to do. Immediate skin-to-skin contact at CS can be very rewarding for many women but may be just too visceral and messy for others.

Postnatal follow-up in these cases is very important. The woman's anxieties may have resolved once the baby is born and she is starting to recover. She may have reflected on what happened and might be feeling better, but there may have been some problems that have provoked a new trauma. Someone trusted, for example her named midwife, should visit her to check whether this is the case. At the same time the midwife will be able to witness the relationship that the woman has with her new baby and make sure that any extra support that she might need is available.

For practical advice on helping women with tokophobia through pregnancy, delivery and the postnatal period, the reader is directed to the Tokophobia Toolkit from the Pan London Perinatal Mental Health Network (Mycroft & Taha 2018).

Mental health issues arising from childbirth

Secondary tokophobia is severe fear of childbirth that arises subsequent to a previous traumatic birth. This can include a miscarriage, a stillbirth and any other version of childbirth trauma, such as a difficult instrumental delivery, an emergency CS or a serious postpartum haemorrhage. It is important to remember that what is perceived as a traumatic birth will vary hugely from one person to another. It is more common in women who are naturally anxious and the prevalence is approximately 14% of women, although there is a variation from one country to another (O'Connell 2017). Secondary tokophobia may not necessarily manifest in pregnancy because women may avoid getting pregnant after their previous experience.

We have previously made the point that traumatic birth is what the patient says it is. When we listen to some women with secondary tokophobia, it is perfectly obvious why anyone would want to avoid a possible repetition of their experiences. Say, for example, a woman had a damaged pelvic floor from a difficult instrumental delivery that had resulted in her baby spending time in the neonatal unit with possible brain injuries. It would only be fair to offer her an elective CS next time and to ensure that she had supportive care from a small number of experienced professionals during her pregnancy. Other women may equally have secondary tokophobia but their story may be considerably less dramatic when viewed from an obstetric perspective. This does not mean their fears should be dismissed: they still require sensitive care and offers of choice regarding the mode of delivery. To be taken seriously regarding fears of giving birth in less obstetrically obvious cases is hugely beneficial for women. They can breathe a sigh of relief and let go of needing to defend their position: someone in a position of power understands.

The points made in the earlier section on primary tokophobia about antenatal, intrapartum and postnatal care are relevant to the management of women with secondary tokophobia. All these women need sympathetic care, ideally from a small number of members of a perinatal mental health team, with the same emphasis on decision-making being centred around the woman, and reference as before to the Tokophobia Toolkit (Mycroft & Taha 2018).

Possible therapies for tokophobia

There are a variety of possible treatments and interventions that have been shown to be of help to some women with a severe fear of childbirth. These include different types of psychotherapy, such as group psycho-education (Rouhe 2014), in which women with primary tokophobia randomised to a psycho-educative group intervention programme with relaxation fared better than their counterparts who had standard antenatal care; cognitive behavioural therapy (CBT), described for example in a Swedish study of women with primary tokophobia by Nieminen et al (2015) and eye movement desensitisation and reprocessing (EMDR) therapy. EMDR is a psychological intervention used for treating those with traumatic memories. It is recognised as a useful treatment for PTSD (NICE 2018) and has been studied as a possible therapy for tokophobia (Bass et al 2017).

These therapies are specialised services and not readily available on the NHS, but where possible it might be worth working with the local mental health services to see what they can offer.

PTSD and postnatal depression

Posttraumatic stress disorder (PTSD) is an anxiety disorder caused by either experiencing or witnessing an event or series of events that have caused fear, distress or shock. Symptoms of PTSD can manifest physically, emotionally or psychologically: they include flashbacks, panic attacks, disturbed sleeping patterns and feelings of violence or complete helplessness. If a woman or her partner develop PTSD following a birth it is a sure sign that the birth was traumatic and their usual ways of coping with stress have been stretched beyond their capacity: the birth was so stressful they have developed a 'disorder'.

Postnatal depression is not the same as PTSD but the symptoms are not dissimilar. Women are likely to have some or all of the following:

- Feeling down, upset or tearful
- Being restless, agitated or irritable
- Not feeling worth anything, feeling guilty for no reason and judging oneself harshly
- Not feeling like there is much to live for
- Feeling alone, isolated and cut off from others
- Feeling everything is pointless
- An inability to enjoy anything
- Having no confidence or self-esteem
- Feeling suicidal
- Not being able to feel connected to the baby or partner

It is really important for postnatal midwives and GPs to be aware of the difference between PTSD and postnatal depression. In the case of postnatal depression it unlikely that the woman will be able to locate any specific reason for her feelings, whereas the woman with PTSD, if asked about her birth experience, will relate it as being traumatic even if she does not use that word.

Women who develop psychiatric illness after childbirth

Postpartum psychosis occurs in approximately 1 in 1,000 births in the UK. It is more likely to affect woman with bipolar disorder, especially bipolar 1 disorder, characterised by having had at least one manic episode lasting a week or more. There is also a higher incidence in women who have previously had postpartum psychosis. Having said that, for many women it happens out of the blue.

The usual onset of postpartum psychosis is within a few days or weeks of giving birth. Women will become excitable, irritated, overly talkative and very confused, and many experience hallucinations and delusions and become paranoid. The delusions may take on a religious nature, such as the belief that the baby is the Devil.

Women with postpartum psychosis will need to be treated in hospital with antipsychotic medication. Some of these medications can be used while breastfeeding, but some may mean that the baby will need to be bottle-fed instead. The Drugs and Lactation database website (LactMed 2006) has very useful information about all types of medication and breastfeeding.

It may take up to 12 months for women with postpartum psychosis to recover, although many will have a reduction in the most severe symptoms after a few weeks. Roughly half of them will develop postpartum psychosis after a future pregnancy and so trying to arrange the right support in advance is hugely important.

The charity Action on Postpartum Psychosis provides an excellent resource for patients and their families on this subject (www.app-network.org).

Pregnant women with pre-existing serious psychiatric illness

Each maternity unit should ideally have a perinatal mental health lead. This will often be a consultant obstetrician or a senior midwife who will liaise with specialist midwives, perinatal psychiatrists, general psychiatrists, mental health nurses and psychologists to provide holistic care for pregnant women with serious psychiatric illness. Women who require this kind of joined-up specialist care will, for example, be detained under the Mental Health Act (MHA) because of severe bipolar or schizo-affective disorder.

Women with severe psychiatric illness are at risk of having a traumatic birth experience unless there has been careful planning beforehand by a good MDT. This must include a specialist mental health midwife with whom the woman has hopefully developed some sort of rapport.

Detention under the MHA does not necessarily mean that the woman is unable to give or refuse consent for obstetric procedures, but her mental capacity may fluctuate. It is wise to try to discuss her wishes for childbirth as early in the pregnancy as possible, during a lucid interval. This means that any plans that need to be made to try to prevent the birth from being traumatic can be discussed and organised well in advance. It is helpful to know, for example, whether she feels that the safety of the baby is an important consideration for her, even if this means having to have an operative delivery.

In the case of a planned CS, the timing of the operation and the personnel to be involved can be carefully arranged in advance, and the operation can take place in a controlled environment that is safe for both the patient and her baby. If the CS is carried out before 38 weeks' gestation, the psychiatrist will probably ask that you do not give steroids for fetal lung maturation (for fear of exacerbating the patient's psychiatric symptoms). You should warn your neonatal colleagues accordingly in case the baby requires admission to the neonatal unit because of respiratory distress.

A series of Best Interest meetings, with contributions from all members of the MDT, should be arranged well in advance of the end of the pregnancy so that plans can be drawn up in good time. If possible one of the patient's close family members should attend at least one of the meetings, and if a family member is not available, the patient should have an independent mental capacity advocate (IMCA) appointed to speak on her behalf.

If an elective CS is planned, in the woman's best interests, this will require agreement from the Court of Protection, which must of course sit well in advance of the due date. Witness statements will be required from members of the MDT for the Court to consider. One person (often, but not always, a consultant obstetrician) from the MDT will be designated as the 'decision maker' and will have to set out clearly the reasons for the MDT's plan and why another plan would not be in the patient's best interests. If the patient ends up needing to be delivered by an emergency CS, no Court agreement is required, but knowledge of this should not be an excuse for 'forgetting' to make a plan for the Court of Protection in the first place.

Pregnant women with serious psychiatric conditions must have specialist midwifery care, and an assessment of capacity must take place as early as possible during the antenatal period. The midwife should aim, if possible, to gain the patient's trust and to maintain it, however challenging this might be, so that the patient's wishes and fears can be conveyed to the MDT and any plans for treatment and delivery can be made in good time.

References

Action on Postpartum Psychosis. www.app-network.org.

Bass M et al. The OptiMUM study: EMDR therapy in pregnant women with posttraumatic stress disorder after previous childbirth and pregnant women with fear of childbirth: Design of a multicentre randomized controlled trial. *European Journal of Psychotraumatology* 2017; 8(1): 1293315. https://www.ncbi.nlm.nih.gov/pmc/articles/PMC5345578/.

LactMed. 2006. Drugs and lactation database. https://www.ncbi.nlm.nih.gov/books/NBK501922/.

Mycroft R, Taha S. Fear of childbirth (Tokophobia) and traumatic experience of childbirth: Best practice toolkit. Healthy London Partnership. 2018. https://www.healthylondon.org/wp-content/uploads/2018/01/Tokophobia-best-practice-toolkit-Jan-2018.pdf.

NICE. Post-traumatic stress disorder. *Guideline NG116*. 5 December 2018.

NICE. Deciding whether to offer caesarean section. 2020. pathways.nice.org.uk.

Nieminen K et al. Nulliparous pregnant women's narratives of imminent childbirth before and after internet-based cognitive behavioural therapy for severe fear of childbirth: A qualitative study. *British Journal of Obstetrics and Gynaecology* 2015; 122(9): 1259–1265.

O'Connell M et al. Worldwide prevalence of tocophobia in pregnant women: Systematic review and meta-analysis. *Acta Obstetricia et Gynecologica Scandinavica* 30 March 2017. https://doi.org/10.1111/aogs.13138.

Rouhe H et al. Group psychoeducation with relaxation for severe fear of childbirth improves maternal adjustment and childbirth experience – a randomised controlled trial. *Journal of Psychosomatic Obstetrics & Gynecology* 2014; 1–9. DOI: 10.3109/0167482X.2014.980722.

Slade P. Establishing a valid construct of fear of childbirth with interviews with women and midwives. *BMC Pregnancy and Childbirth* 2019; 19(1): 96. https://bmcpregnancychildbirth.biomedcentral.com/articles/10.1186/s12884-019-2241-7.

Sperlich M et al. Integrating trauma-informed care into maternity care practice: Conceptual and practical issues. *Journal Midwifery & Women's Health* 2017; 62: 661–672.

Wright M. Psychological and physiological impacts of child sexual abuse during pregnancy, birth and postnatally. Narrowcast Media Group. Vimeo. 5 February 2019.

10 Debriefing and Serious Incident reporting

The Oxford Dictionary definition of the word 'debrief' is 'a series of questions about a completed mission or undertaking'. The term has its origins in the military world and may be used in the context of extracting information from spies. The medical use of the word involves giving as well as getting accurate information, hopefully in a rather less aggressive manner.

It is not unusual for a birth plan to contain a phrase that is something like 'please inform me about what is happening and about what you are going to do to me'. This should go without saying: of course, doctors and midwives would not do something to a woman without talking to her about it, would they? And yet many women do not understand what happened to them during their labour and delivery, especially if it did not go according to plan, and they will have many questions to ask and comments to make afterwards. It is fair to say that a woman's memories of labour and delivery could be clouded by a variety of factors: painkilling drugs, tiredness, a certain protective mechanism in the brain that blots out the details of anything that was difficult or painful. It is important for the staff to understand this and to be prepared to explain what happened, not just once, at the time, but again after the event, when the woman is in a better position to retain the information and to ask the questions she wants to ask.

Debriefing for patients

It would be normal practice for a doctor to talk to a woman immediately after an emergency CS to reassure her that all is well and to tell her the basics of what had happened. The doctor might say something like 'we had to deliver the baby this way because he was in the wrong position, with his head looking upwards instead of downwards, and so he got himself stuck. I'm pleased to say that he's fine and the operation went well. You didn't lose very much blood and you should heal up with no problems'. The doctor can then tick the box marked 'debrief' in the notes and feel satisfied with a job well done.

If the mother is in a fit state a little later, it might also be helpful to ask her how much of what happened she understood at the time, whether she felt she had been included in the decision to do the best thing for her baby or whether she felt ignored in the immediacy of her needing a CS. Doing this will help her to feel that her experience of events mattered. If there really was no time to include her preferences due the emergency, understanding her perspective will inform you about her state of mind. Understanding why something is being done, or retrospectively, why an action was taken, can help people process events. If she is not in a fit state to talk (and therefore not a fit state to listen) reassure her that you will see her again.

The next day, on the postnatal ward round, it would be very helpful if a doctor (preferably the same one who did the operation) went through the details of that explanation again, when the woman has had a chance to begin to come to terms with what happened to her and is in a position to ask questions. It might help to have a doll and a pelvis in the postnatal ward to help with the explanation, especially if the cause of the problem was a malposition, and a sheet of paper in case drawing a picture would add to the discussion. The woman might think that the malposition was her fault (either wittingly, because she wasn't pushing hard enough, or unwittingly, because of some misshapen part of her pelvis that hadn't been detected before) and this would be a good opportunity to reassure her that neither was the case. She might remember some of what had been said to her immediately after the operation but it is best to assume that she knows nothing and to start again from the beginning. Tell her that you are beginning again because you are not sure how much she remembers.

Good practice with regard to this debrief would also include a written version to be given to the woman before she is discharged from hospital, with a copy, either electronic or on paper, on the GP's discharge summary. By doing this both the woman and her GP have an accurate version of events, which is helpful if she has further questions at the time of her six week check-up with the GP, or if she wants to book at another unit in a future pregnancy.

More often than not, the day 1 debrief is done by a junior doctor who was not present at the delivery and who lacks the experience to be able to answer any question that is at all complicated. He or she will be able to read the operation notes and repeat them to the woman, but may not be able to go much further than that. Staffing rotas in a maternity unit need to recognise that the postnatal ward is a place where more senior members of staff are required.

Sometimes (many times?) none of this happens, or if it does, it often happens in a way that means that the woman either doesn't understand the explanation or doesn't remember it. If this does not happen, then unless the woman or her birth partner make it obvious that they need to discuss their birth experience there will be no opportunity for them to review the birth and come to an understanding about it. Questions about the birth may surface unexpectedly during a consultation about something else, or may not arise until the next pregnancy when someone asks about her choice of mode of delivery. It is not uncommon for an obstetrician or midwife to go through the old hospital notes during an antenatal appointment to see what had happened during the last delivery and to explain this to the woman, often in the spirit of helping her to decide about how to deliver this time. Say, for example, the previous baby weighed 4 kg and was in a deflexed occipito–posterior (OP) position, and the CS was for failure to progress in the first stage of labour. One might say that if this baby seems to be the same sort of size as the previous one, it might be better to plan to do another CS, but that if this one looked smaller and was in an appropriate position it would be worth trying to deliver normally. The woman may have known that the previous CS was due to the baby's size and position, but at times it is as if she is hearing this information for the first time. The consultation is marked by the sound of pennies dropping: 'oh, so *that's* why he wouldn't come out'. It is unlikely that the staff at the time failed to talk to the woman about her delivery, but she has not remembered what they said to her or what it meant. Alternatively, the explanation was given from the medical staff's point of view and she did not feel she could speak about her understanding or lack of it.

What if the details of the delivery are more worrying? Giving difficult information almost in real time is a challenge but it must be done clearly and honestly. Taking the example of an emergency CS again, what if, for instance, there was excessive bleeding, unexpected damage to the woman's bladder, and the baby has had to go to the neonatal unit because he was having trouble breathing? This time the obstetrician has to say something like 'we had to deliver the baby by Caesarean section because he was in the wrong position, with his head looking upwards instead of downwards, and so he got himself stuck. I don't think anyone really knew about this until you had been in labour for a long time. Because he was stuck and it was a bit tricky to deliver him, he has developed some problems with his breathing and our colleagues in the special care baby unit are looking after him for a while until he is able to breathe on his own. You lost a lot of blood during the Caesarean and because of this it was more difficult than usual to repair your womb. We're giving you some blood now to make up for the blood that you lost. Your bladder was damaged during the operation but we have repaired it, although you will need to have a catheter in for the next 10 days so that your bladder can rest and recover. I'm sorry this is all so complicated but I'll come back to see you again in a little while and I'll be able to answer any questions'. It would be useful to acknowledge at this point what a hard time she and her partner have had and that they are likely to worried about their baby, and if possible, you should tell them when they will be able to go and see him. If that is not possible at the moment, then ensure that someone from the neonatal unit comes to see them soon.

These three major problems (blood loss from uterine atony, bladder damage, a hypoxic baby requiring neonatal unit admission) are not totally unexpected in the context of an obstructed labour, which is why obstetricians need to be alert to the signs of the labour becoming obstructed so that if possible, complications like these can be averted.

Whilst we can quote the incidence of each of these complications arising from an emergency CS, it is important that we remember that the woman's pregnancy journey started with an expectation that she would have a normal delivery and that all with be well with her and her baby. Her impression at the start of the process would have been that the risk of any of these things happening to her would be very small, let alone the risk of all three happening at once. Each one is difficult to contemplate and each will jostle for position in her mind ('I've had to have a blood transfusion; my bladder may not work properly again and I might be incontinent; my baby is in special care on a breathing machine and he might have brain damage'). This is also a very challenging time for her partner, who will have to oscillate between the recovery room to be with her and the neonatal unit to be with the baby.

A promise to return to answer questions ('I'll come back to see you again in a little while and I'll be able to answer any questions') *must* be kept. If you have made that promise and you are unexpectedly delayed by another emergency, you must pass a message to the member of staff looking after the woman to say that you have been held up but that you will be back later, with a reasonable estimate of when that might be. When you return you must be prepared to spend time with the woman and her partner, so get your other tasks done first so that as far as possible you can talk to them without interruption. You will need to be honest about what has happened and about what they should expect in the next 12–24 hours, and you should apologise if in any way the management could be criticised (if, for example, there were signs of obstructed labour for some hours prior to the delivery that were not recognised or not acknowledged as being serious).

The Duty of Candour rules (CQC 2014) mean that there is a statutory duty to be open and honest with patients when something goes wrong. In the past staff were not encouraged to be honest and say sorry for fear of litigation, but now not only is it good manners but it is a legal requirement.

Hopefully a member of staff from the neonatal unit will have already talked to the couple about the baby's condition and about what the next few hours might bring. If they have not done so, you should go and find out what is happening to the baby and report back to the parents in simple terms, with a promise that your neonatal colleague will be along as soon as they can, to explain things in more detail. If it is possible, get a commitment from your neonatal colleague as to when they will visit. This will help contain the understandable anxiety the parents will be experiencing. It is especially important if the baby's condition is very serious and if the neonatal staff are considering transferring the baby to another unit for further treatment such as therapeutic cooling. If the baby is going to be transferred to another hospital, you should, if possible, ensure that the mother is sufficiently stable to be transferred to the same place, and you should talk to the obstetric consultant on call there to ensure that they will be able to accommodate her.

These paragraphs have discussed the importance of explaining what happened, which is distinct from counselling the parents about what happened. They are different processes but both need to happen.

The descriptions given here are graphic and it is likely that staff will realise that the couple has had a traumatic experience and that they need immediate help to take in what has happened, and might need ongoing support to deal with the aftermath of their ordeal. Counselling within a Women's Health department should be available for them both.

If possible, a counsellor will meet the parents whilst they are still in hospital, as one of the jobs a counsellor may take on, on their behalf, is to be an advocate. The bewilderment felt after a trauma sometimes makes it hard for parents to know what to expect, let alone know who they can or should speak to about their concerns. This situation can be eased by a member staff who has the role of advocate. Additionally, appointments can be offered to see both or one of the parents in a safe place away from the ward, where emotions can be expressed and queries and questions can be explored. It is a counsellor's job to be there in a non-judgemental, empathic manner whilst people recover their physical and emotional health.

Debriefing for staff

Occasionally a case is so unusually difficult or shocking that the staff involved are shaken by what has happened and require a debrief of their own. For this to be effective it should be done fairly soon after the event, with as many of the staff involved as possible gathered in one place, and with the session led by someone who can facilitate a discussion that is inclusive and non-judgemental. I remember this taking place after a case just before Christmas of a concealed pregnancy that turned into shoulder dystocia involving an infant that had suffered an intrauterine death. The delivery took place in theatre so that the mother could be anaesthetised and the theatre staff, who were used to difficult deliveries but not used to stillbirths, found it very unsettling. We arranged for all those involved to meet and talk about what happened, and I was struck by how much the theatre team seemed to appreciate the fact that the obstetrician delivering the baby had found it difficult too, and that we were all human after all.

Just as we know that many births are not recognised as being traumatic for mothers, it may well be that staff are also dealing with distress regarding less obviously harrowing births. A culture for being able to speak about how one is affected by stress has not really existed until very recently. It is likely to have been seen as a sign of weakness, or people feared that it was. The example stated here illustrates how relieved staff were to discover that the obstetrician had similar feelings to them – without the obstetrician saying so, the theatre staff may have stayed silent. Coping mechanisms, where we try to carry on regardless, deny us the opportunity to trust our own experiences. If something was tough to experience when dealing with patients it is not healthy to deny it, nor is it healthy to blame patients. As mentioned in the chapter on being a patient and person-centred care, Schwartz Rounds are trying to break through the barriers of shame and shyness regarding the cost of caring. As well as these formalised gatherings where feelings can be expressed, we should try to enable our colleagues to feel that they can talk about how they have been affected by their work and have systems in place to provide help and support for those who need it.

A formal debrief for parents after the event

In cases that are sufficiently serious or complicated, then a formal debrief meeting should be offered after the event, once the woman has recovered physically and been discharged from the hospital. The meeting should be arranged before she leaves the hospital if possible, or if not then, soon after she has gone home, so that she knows the date and can make her domestic arrangements. If the baby has been discharged from the hospital, she will need to arrange for someone to look after him or her at home or to come to the hospital with her so that the baby can be cared for whilst she attends the meeting. She will probably bring her partner with her, and perhaps someone else, a friend or relative, whom she trusts to remember what is said and to ask the questions that she has forgotten.

Ideally her named consultant will be present at the meeting, especially if he or she was involved clinically in the woman's case, as they will be best placed to explain the details of what happened and to answer questions. It is good practice not to do this alone, and the other attendees could include a senior midwife, or someone from the hospital's risk office or Patient Advisory Liaison Service (PALS). This is useful especially since the case may be the subject of a formal complaint and the PALS team may already be aware of it. If the mother has been receiving counselling, she may want the counsellor to be present as well.

The consultant must be well prepared for the meeting, having read the notes carefully first and made a summary of the main points to be covered. Likely questions and issues of concern should be anticipated and thought through beforehand so that they do not come as a surprise when mentioned by the woman or one of her relatives. Other colleagues may be included in the meeting if the case warrants their presence – for example, a neonatologist if the baby required complex treatment in the neonatal unit.

The meeting room should be booked for three hours, with refreshments (at least glasses of water, preferably tea and coffee) provided. There should be at least a 15-minute pre-meeting in an adjacent room so that the staff can talk about the main points they think will be discussed and make sure that each knows the others' views about them. The meeting itself will require up to two hours, and the timing should be made clear from the start when the woman and her relatives arrive – 'we have two hours set aside for this meeting' – so that they do not feel as if they are going to be hurried out. If at the end of the two hours it is obvious a further meeting is required, the attendees can be assured that this will be arranged in a timely fashion. There should then be time allowed after the meeting, once the woman has left, for the staff to consider what has been said and make plans about who is going to do what.

The meeting will be recorded and the woman may be offered a copy of the recording on a CD. Some women may also record the meeting themselves on a mobile phone and they have every right to do so. Staff members must accept from the start that this is going to happen and choose their words accordingly. Women will also want a copy of the hospital notes if they haven't already been given a copy. Some hospitals request a nominal sum of money for photocopying the notes, but in the context of a difficult case this seems petty and it would be polite to waive the charge.

Parents and their relatives may understandably become emotional during the meeting and the staff members present must accept that this will happen. Staff should keep their own emotions under control, without coming across as unfeeling or callous.

A written summary of the points covered in the meeting must be sent to the woman within a few days of the meeting, with a copy to her GP. It is good practice to make it clear at the start of the meeting that this will happen so that she does not think that she will have to remember absolutely everything that is said to her. The letter, of course, must be completely honest, should include an apology if one is warranted and should contain contact details in case there are further questions.

After the meeting the staff involved will need time to make notes about any particular details that will need to be covered in the summary letter. They may also need to consider whether further advice or action is needed from someone else (say, a urologist if there are ongoing symptoms arising from bladder damage). They should, if possible, not go straight to their next clinic/meeting/operating list, but instead allow themselves some time to reflect about what was said in the meeting. This is good practice in relation to looking after oneself.

Serious Incident reporting

Clinical incidents should be reported immediately and if they are of sufficient gravity they will be declared as a Serious Incident (SI) very soon after this. Statements will be obtained from the staff members involved and an investigating team will carry out a root cause analysis and write a report. The team will comprise senior staff members who had no clinical involvement in the case. Incidents involving a maternal death, an intrapartum stillbirth, an early neonatal death or severe hypoxic ischaemic encephalopathy will be investigated by the external Healthcare Safety Investigation Branch (HSIB) but many Trusts will still carry out their own review of these cases as well.

An incident will appear different depending on who is looking at it. Those involved in the incident itself will each have their take on the matter, and each will believe that what they saw/did/witnessed is the truth. In fact, the whole story can only be told by someone who is able to glean the opinions of each of the people involved, and who then by piecing the information gathered together can come up with a reasonably coherent whole. Just as when a number of people look at a scene and then describe it, each remembering different things, so it is with a clinical incident, when each person has their view of part of the incident but cannot see the whole picture. An independent investigator (usually, but not always, a consultant obstetrician and/or a senior midwife) will gather information from all those involved and put it together in a way that each of those contributing could not possibly do, and in a way that hopefully makes sense, even if that sense is complicated or upsetting.

An example of 'only telling part of the story' can arise if the investigator does not make enquiries about the context of the incident – in other words, what else was going on at the time. If something went wrong because a doctor didn't attend to a labouring woman in time, it could be construed that the doctor was neglecting her. In fact, the doctor may well have been busy with another emergency case, and could not have been expected to be in two places at once. Only by finding out the whole story can a correct narrative be constructed. In this case, for example, the summary would not be 'the doctor should have been there and because he/she wasn't, he/she was to blame for what went wrong' but 'the doctor should have been there, but he/she was having to deal with another case at the same time: in order to prevent a repeat of incidents like this we need to have more senior staff on duty'.

Another example is when the same incident is seen differently by those immediately involved. One example of this is a case in which a woman needed an emergency CS because she was hyponatraemic and the baby's CTG showed signs of hypoxia. Because of her condition the woman was delirious and in no state to sign a consent form. The obstetric team took her to theatre and wanted to get on with the CS, but there was a delay whilst the theatre team questioned the absence of a consent form. In the end the obstetrician found consent form 4, which allows a doctor to proceed in someone's best interests when they cannot consent for themselves, and the CS went ahead. The case was declared a Serious Incident (SI) because the baby was hypoxic at birth and had to be admitted to the neonatal unit. There were initial worries at the time about the theatre team delaying the CS, but the SI investigator discovered that all the theatre staff had had a teaching session earlier that week by the legal team about the importance of the correct use of the different types of consent forms. They were right to question the absence of a consent form, and the obstetricians could have prevented the delay by completing consent form 4 in the first place while the patient was being wheeled to the operating theatre.

It can be challenging to investigate an incident and then write a comprehensive, truthful report. You will not necessarily endear yourself to those involved when you tell it like it is and your duty to tell the truth may make you unpopular with some within the hospital management who might prefer the report to be bland rather than critical. Although senior managers now recognise the importance of duty of candour in principle, they also have at least one eye on the lawyers who are likely to use a SI report as evidence of liability. But if you are going to write a SI report properly you must tell the truth, warts and all, and not shy away from explaining what went wrong and why and drawing critical conclusions if these are appropriate.

The language of the report is important because of the variety of people who will be reading it, including the patient to whom it relates, and her family. It is primarily a document for the Trust, but it will be shared amongst a number of other people including members of the Clinical Commissioning Group and NHS Resolution (formerly known as the rather harsher sounding NHS Litigation Authority). For this reason, it should be written in non-medical language as much as possible, with a glossary to explain abbreviations or unavoidable medical terms. The personnel are not named but ascribed a code-name (doctor 1, midwife 2, for example) to preserve their anonymity, but the author of the report will of course be able to identify who was who. A draft copy must be sent to the staff members who provided the statements before the report is finalised so that they can check for factual accuracy.

The report should be completed six weeks after the SI was declared, and then, once it has been signed by the Trust's Chief Executive, it should be shared amongst the relevant parties including the members of staff directly involved with the case and with the patient/parents. It should be sent to them with a covering letter to explain why it has been written, and offering a meeting with the report's author or authors so that the findings can be discussed. This meeting is separate from and different to any meeting to discuss the clinical aspects of the case.

During the meeting to discuss the report and its findings, the parents may want to know what has happened to the staff involved – are they still at work? Have they been suspended? It can be a challenge explaining that the features of the case were such that no one individual was actually at fault and that all the members of staff concerned are continuing to work. Even if the conclusion of the investigation was that the incident arose because of the fault of a particular member of staff, the recommendation may well be that this person is suspended temporarily pending extra training, rather than sacked. When the consequence of the 'incident' is catastrophic to parents and their families, e.g. their baby died or will be disabled for the rest of their, perhaps shortened, life, it can be very difficult for them to understand how, if someone is accountable, they can keep their job.

In our experience being honest and open with parents when something has gone wrong can sometimes have a profound effect. They change from feeling hostile and defensive to feeling understood and that their perspective has been included.

When an apology by a Trust is needed, it is really important not to be insulting to the recipients. For example, it is very different to receive an apology like 'I am sorry I kicked you' from an apology that says 'I am sorry you felt hurt when I kicked you'. The former apologises for the actual act and it implies ownership of the wrongdoing, whilst the latter implies that it is the patient's interpretation or reaction that is being apologised for. Patients can tell when individuals or institutions are being sincere and when they are not.

The SI report's authors are also responsible for checking that any action points arising from the case are carried out in the specified time frame. This can be a challenge if the recommendations (e.g. provide more midwives on the labour ward on the night shifts) are at odds with the Trust's spending plans, and the report's authors will need support from their Clinical and Divisional Directors in relation to this.

Reference

CQC. Health and social care act 2008 (Regulated Activities) regulations 2014: Regulation 20: Duty of Candour. 2014.

11 Managing the next pregnancy and delivery

A debrief after a traumatic birth

The management of the next pregnancy begins immediately after the traumatic birth itself, with a clear and truthful account of what happened, what had to be done and what all that means for the future. This is discussed in detail in the chapter on debriefing. Any explanation given soon after a traumatic birth will need to be repeated, as the woman will be in no position to remember everything that is said to her at the time. Ideally, she should also be given something in writing explaining the details, either before she leaves the hospital or soon after she has been discharged, with a copy sent to her GP. Our experience is that mothers and their partners are keen to have cast-iron plans in place regarding their next pregnancy and delivery. Knowing that staff understand and care about their previous experience and that as much as possible will be done to avoid a repeat of their previous experience is a huge relief.

After a traumatic birth, patients may ask 'will I be able to get pregnant again?' or 'will I be able to have another baby?' It would be very unusual for the answer to those questions to be 'no': this would be the case if she had had to have an emergency hysterectomy, which is discussed in the chapter on surgical considerations. For the majority of patients the answer will be 'yes', or 'yes, when you both feel ready' or 'yes, bearing in mind these caveats'.

'When you both feel ready'

This comment can sometimes instigate a difficult conversation. For some couples this is a simple decision: they are very clear that they want to be pregnant again as soon as possible, as if to prove to themselves and others that 'they can do it'. Other couples will be equally clear that they do not want to get pregnant again straightaway and will want to have a break from the pressure of pregnancy for a while. They may even ask your advice about contraception. In the circumstances this is entirely understandable: it does not take much imagination to appreciate how scared the woman may feel about having another baby, and even if she isn't scared, her partner will doubtless feel very scared having witnessed everything that went on when the birth was traumatic.

The discussion becomes more complicated if one of them feels differently from the other. The woman may be very anxious to be pregnant again but her partner may feel equally anxious about avoiding another pregnancy because their recent experience was so terrifying. In other cases these feelings may be reversed: the partner is keen to try for another baby but the woman is afraid and self-protective, not wanting to risk something so awful happening to her again.

This is a challenging situation for a couple to find themselves in and it may be that counselling can help them explore their feelings. The role of the counsellor would be to help each of them have a voice without taking sides. It may be that being together in a safe place, they can talk about what happened to them during the trauma of the birth and that they will reach an understanding of each other. As a consequence, one of them can perhaps shift their position and agree to either try for another baby or limit their family to the size it currently is. However, this may not be the case: some couples cannot reach an understanding of each other and they remain separated in their own positions. Some couples will handle this and remain together. One person will give in to the other person's perception. They may still disagree and remain a couple, even if it means bearing some resentment towards each other, each feeling 'if only they would see my point of view'. Other relationships may break down, because the consequences of the other not being able to understand and the consequences of there being another pregnancy or not is too much pressure for the couple.

'Yes, bearing in mind these caveats'

Possible caveats would be:

- Ideally you should wait a few months before trying again, until your blood pressure is under control.
- Ideally you should wait a few months before trying again, so that you can have tests to make sure the repair of your tear has been effective.
- You would need to be delivered by a planned CS in the future.
- You would need to be delivered by a planned CS in the future and this must be done by an experienced consultant because you are likely to have adhesions.

All of these topics can be discussed in as much detail as the couple needs, and the points documented so that staff in the future are fully aware of any arrangements that will need to be made.

Consider a preconceptual appointment

Some patients will be so affected by their previous pregnancy experience that they will not consider getting pregnant again until they have had some form of reassurance about how the pregnancy and delivery will be managed. This may be true despite a debrief regarding the previous pregnancy having taken place. It is of course impossible to guarantee that all will be well the next time, and it would be foolish to pretend that the next pregnancy will be completely trouble-free, but it can be helpful to go over some practical points so that the patient has at least got some sort of structure on which to hang her thoughts. For women who have had a traumatic birth, the thought of another pregnancy might be terrifying, and if they felt that the next pregnancy was a step into the unknown, the terror would be even more severe. If on the other hand they knew roughly what would happen and when, they can begin to consider how they would manage and what they would have to do in order to cope with their fears and keep them under some sort of control. At a preconceptual meeting they can also find out how they will be supported and aided, and how care will be given which might go some way towards alleviating any specific fears.

Some patients will have medical reasons for needing a preconceptual clinic appointment – for example, those with high blood pressure or brittle diabetes – and having a review prior to the next pregnancy would be a matter of routine. Women who have had a traumatic birth will not necessarily fit into a 'medical' category but will warrant a careful discussion about how a future pregnancy will be managed, with the same amount of attention to detail: a 'pregnancy plan', if you will. This might include the following:

- Addressing any medical issues such as blood pressure control, if necessary
- Discussing whether she will book for antenatal care via her GP as usual or whether she will get in touch with the hospital obstetrician or midwife directly, with the relevant contact details
- Whether she wants her antenatal care to be at the same hospital or whether she would prefer to go somewhere else
- A schedule for antenatal appointments and scans
- A schedule for counselling appointments, taking into consideration relevant dates (for example, if she has previously suffered a 22-week pregnancy loss, she will need extra support when she approaches the same gestation in the coming pregnancy)
- A provisional plan about mode and timing of delivery, bearing in mind that the clinical situation might dictate a change in these arrangements

Having some knowledge of what will happen in advance once she is pregnant again can be very helpful for some women who have suffered a traumatic birth. I remember one woman who had a very preterm delivery associated with chorioamnionitis, and her baby lived for only a few days afterwards. The neonatal doctors realised that the baby was not going to survive and talked to her and her partner about turning off the ventilator to let him die. She understood the logic of this but was not able to let the doctors take that final step until she knew how a future pregnancy would be managed. A meeting in the neonatal office was hastily arranged and we went through what would happen, in principle, when she was pregnant again – regular care from a small number of people; swabs to check for infection; possible prophylactic antibiotics; an increased number of scans for reassurance. Only once she had had that conversation was she able to let the doctors turn off the machines and say goodbye to her baby, knowing how his future brother or sister might be protected.

Read the notes

If you are to help her in the next pregnancy, it is vital that you understand the details of what happened in the mother's previous pregnancy and delivery. You want to be able to cut to the chase when you see her at her antenatal appointments, so that she does not have to repeat parts of her story and does not need to remind you about some piece of information that you have forgotten. You should both be able to begin where you left off at the last antenatal appointment, remembering what was said before and moving on to what needs to be said now.

Failure to read the notes first can make for clumsy mistakes and horrible 'foot in mouth' encounters. 'So this is your second baby, yes? And how old is your first? Oh, I see, I'm so sorry. . .' when a look at her notes will tell you that her first baby was stillborn following an abruption. This is the case for everyone with whom the woman comes into contact, so if you have any influence over the appointments system you must try to limit the number of people she sees as much as possible and make sure that those who have been trusted with her care are aware of her story. Ideally this small number of trusted individuals will comprise a midwife, a sonographer and an obstetrician. With a bit of forward planning you can do your best to organise appointments so that she only sees these three people for all her antenatal visits. We cannot overstate how beneficial this kind of care can be. It is hugely reassuring and can to some extent mitigate any lasting effects of the previous trauma. It helps ensure that the woman and her partner are not left floundering in the aftermath of their earlier ordeal. They can put their trust in the care they receive if it is limited to a small number of people and those people are consistent in their care.

Members of staff can easily make mistakes when they fail to read the notes properly. I remember a patient who had had a CS for her first delivery because of fetal distress, and who had since grown a very large fibroid in the lower part of her uterus, which blocked the way out for the second baby, who had to lie in a transverse position. She was seen in the antenatal clinic by a junior doctor who had been taught the mantra of ensuring that women with one previous CS were encouraged to have a VBAC the next time, and who insisted to this woman that she should deliver normally. Cue her tears, a complaint, a hastily arranged appointment with a consultant (who had read the notes) and the scheduling of her CS. What should have been a relatively straightforward encounter turned unnecessarily into a drama that the woman could have done without. One excuse for this kind of mistake is that the clinics are very busy, but clinics become busier still if members of staff don't read the notes before they speak and then have to arrange extra appointments to make up for what went wrong.

Not everyone with whom the woman comes into contact will be able to read the notes, making it the responsibility of the person in charge of the case to convey the relevant information to the right people beforehand. For example, if the woman is due to deliver normally but there are important aspects of her history that colleagues should know, these can be shared by email ahead of her due date so that everyone who should know about her is aware of the issues surrounding her case. Similarly, if a woman with a difficult obstetric history is due to have a planned CS, these details can be shared with the theatre staff during the 'team-briefing' session before the operating list begins. 'Team-briefing' is a structured introduction session prior to the commencement of an operating list to ensure that all the members of staff know each other and that the details of each case are discussed and agreed in advance (http://www.nrls.npsa.nhs.uk). This means that everyone knows the basic facts about what happened to the woman previously and no one makes any unwittingly crass remarks or asks any unwanted questions.

Arrange a visit

Some women who have had a traumatic birth will be very worried about revisiting the scene and will be anxious about the possibility of being in the same labour room again, or of having to revisit the same operating theatre. Some will welcome the opportunity to be accompanied on a visit to the labour ward as the due date approaches, so that they can become somewhat desensitised and its horrors can be put into some sort of perspective. It is obviously difficult to engineer a quiet labour ward day for the visit, and you may need to be flexible about timings and about which rooms you can go into, but it is worth making the effort for people who are scared.

We did this for a couple whose first child had suffered a neonatal death following a difficult instrumental delivery. They were due to have a planned CS but were frightened about the prospect of being in the operating theatre again. We took them on a tour of the labour ward during a relatively peaceful time, and we showed them the empty operating theatre so that we could explain what was what (the anaesthetic machine, the resuscitaire, and so on) and who would be where on the day. They were able to feel scared in a protected way during that visit, and when the day of the actual CS arrived, they felt calmer than they had expected as a result. It was also a way of honouring the enormity of the death of their son: we were acknowledging that the last time they were on the labour ward they were full of sorrow. We wanted them to be prepared for the birth of their second baby without being overwhelmed by painful memories.

Planning the delivery

There will be those who feel that the only way to deal with the memory of a previous traumatic birth, whatever form the trauma took, would be to have a planned CS next time. Even if there was no serious perineal damage, or if any uterine scarring was such that a VBAC would be a reasonable option, women may feel that the only thing to do would be to have a CS. They are likely to be supported in this notion by family and friends and it would be difficult to argue with her. Others will want to deliver normally, especially if they had wanted to do this the first time and couldn't, or if they had delivered normally last time and the trauma they experienced was related to something else.

A planned CS has the advantage of being relatively easy to organise and gives everyone a more or less predictable plan, with a date in the diary and an expectation that everything will be under control. A woman who wants a spontaneous onset of labour and a normal delivery will have accepted that nature is in control rather than anyone else, and the onus will be upon her midwife and consultant to make sure that those involved are prepared for her, whatever time of day or night she turns up.

Some women will be so anxious about the prospect of waiting for the due date that they will want to be delivered early. This is commonly the case for those who have had a previous stillbirth or neonatal death: the thought of going to term and 'pushing their luck' is too much to bear. If after a discussion there is a plan for an early delivery, she may need to be given steroids to aid fetal lung maturation and, depending on the gestation, the neonatal team may need to be informed about the plan.

The delivery

There are some fairly simple considerations that can make the arrangements go more smoothly. If a normal delivery is planned, you can make sure the labour ward or birth centre team are aware of the woman and her story, so that the staff are prepared for her whenever she arrives and can give her the care and attention that she needs. This can be by a group email and, if necessary, a personal discussion with the labour ward matron or birth centre manager.

If she is to have a planned CS, then again the relevant staff can be forewarned so that the arrangements on the day run smoothly. The team briefing mentioned earlier will ensure that the theatre staff are aware of the case and know what is expected of them. It would also be wise to arrange for the woman to have a single room once the baby is born, so that her partner can stay with her and she can have some privacy away from the rest of the ward.

You should consider carefully whether you are going to be personally involved (for example, you may have promised to do the CS yourself) or whether a colleague is going to do the procedure instead. There are pros and cons of personal involvement: some couples cling fast to the person they know and feel even more anxious if they have to deal with someone else. On the other hand, last minute changes in the plan may have to be arranged – you may be struck down by illness on the day, for example, and be unable to come to work – and it is also helpful if parents can be gently nudged towards believing that they can trust other people as well as you. Some doctors feel very proud about being in demand and revel in the feeling of being the only person who can look after certain patients, but this is not a sustainable situation. One day you might be unwell, or have an accident on the way to work, or you might be held up by an emergency, and your patients will have to be looked after by someone else. In the end it will be better for them, and for you, if they learn that it is not only you that is capable of caring for them and that they will be in safe hands with one of your colleagues. Anticipating the possibility of your absence by introducing your colleague or a small number of your colleagues to patients is advisable. If this is impossible, you still need to ensure that your colleagues are fully informed about the patient's circumstances so that the impact of your absence is lessened.

Reference

Five steps to safer surgery. 2010. http://www.nrls.npsa.nhs.uk/EasySiteWeb/getresource.axd?AssetID=
    93286.

12 Trauma for staff

Trauma to staff – how does it feel

Experiencing trauma due to an event at work is completely understandable; if the birth of a baby is not as expected and dramatic events happen, it is not only the mother and her partner who will be affected. Due to the roles each member of staff takes during the 'drama' to get the job done, it is unlikely that they will initially have much time to process their reactions or be aware of any lasting impact on them. This does not stop people thinking about how frightened they are during and after the event. They may find themselves wondering if they will be blamed, if they have handled and are handling matters in the best way possible and they may be metaphorically keeping their fingers crossed that all will be well.

It is crucial that staff are given support and guidance as a matter of course and not left to their own devices to cope. If there is no inbuilt structure to care for staff who have suffered in the course of their work, then, often, people will blame themselves when there may be nothing to blame themselves for. They may struggle and doubt their competence, mistaking the concerns they have about their performance as real rather than an attempt to make sense of what happened and what, if anything, went wrong. Conscientious staff will question their part in any event and they need to be able to discuss with the other people involved what happened and to fit the pieces of the whole together. In doing this they may discover that in fact nothing went wrong; that what happened was inevitable. Alternatively, they may discover that something did go wrong and there were interventions that could have made a difference – though this may only become clear retrospectively. We have often remarked that hindsight is a wonderful thing. This is not to excuse any incompetence; if mistakes happened which were avoidable or because of someone's negligence, then people need to be held accountable and given opportunities to learn from their mistakes.

Without support, staff are left to make of traumatic events what they can. For all intents and purposes they may seem to others as if they are unaffected. However, within themselves they feel scared and a 'mess'. They may find themselves avoiding certain situations or individuals that they associate with the original cause of the trauma. It is likely that they will try to side-step work which has any hint of a repetition.

One midwife revealed in a training session, where she felt safe, that she had crossed the road when she saw the mother of a baby who had died at birth. She felt inadequate and did not know what to say: this was despite the fact that she had been helpful at the time of the baby's death. This was some considerable time after the event but her avoidance of something painful had stayed with her. It was not until she had the opportunity of attending sessions designed to help midwives manage pregnancy loss that she could begin to understand why she behaved in the way she did.

Ruth has made reference in the birth plans chapter to the professor who would not or, more correctly, could not allow a Ventouse to be used by his team because of a previous bad experience. This was presumably years after his original trauma and clearly demonstrates that without sufficient support individuals use avoidance tactics to manage their fear. They try to ensure that they never re-experience the original distress, and in his case, he was unable to believe that others could successfully deliver a baby using a Ventouse.

Without adequate support individuals never go through the barrier of fear to discover that they can deal with the horrendous events. In fact, they never learn that they have had a completely normal and appropriate reaction to something terrifying. Left to their own devices, they have to create a way of dealing with the trauma that is inevitable within medicine.

We have learnt in our work with women who have had traumatic births and those who have had a baby die that, if given appropriate care in a subsequent pregnancy, they can separate one horrendous incident from a frightening but ultimately successful experience. They are able to contain their initial hurt in the context of having something positive to contrast with the original pain or sorrow. Each individual and her loved ones can be given that opportunity by ensuring they are looked after according to their separate needs. This is not the case for staff: they need to go on working with many women who have a multitude of health issues. Staff must 'bite the bullet' and many times be frightened that the horrendous outcome will occur again, feeling lucky if it does not. Living in this kind of isolation, where fear and the aftermath of trauma is down to the individual to process, is not healthy. We need to enable staff to feel safe, and that includes feeling safe even when a competent person makes a mistake that has dreadful outcomes.

We will never know whether the professor who avoided the Ventouse was offered help, whether he kept his feelings and reactions to himself, whether he blamed himself or someone more senior than him. What we do know is that he was terrified by his ordeal and made sure he never ever was in danger of a similar experience again.

Obstetrics is inherently complicated and cases can become very serious. It is the nature of the specialty. It takes time for staff to acknowledge this and unless they do, they will feel personally responsible when something bad happens. Senior staff need to support less experienced colleagues about the reason for Serious Incident investigations and help them develop some resilience. This resilience may be hard won because of the level of responsibility midwives, doctors and nurses carry in the course of their working lives. In most occupations, if someone makes a mistake, the consequences are not likely to lead to death or have life-changing aftereffects. This is not the case in maternity services.

Investigations into serious outcomes take place to find out what if anything went wrong, to establish individual responsibility for the various events and to piece the whole 'picture' together. Should the investigation establish that despite each person doing the correct thing at the right time, and the terrible event was inevitable, there should be no blame attached any one individual. Lessons may be learnt and at the same time it is important that senior staff ensure that they find out how each staff member involved is feeling. No blame does not mean that people are not traumatised.

If the investigation uncovers errors made by any one person or a number of people, it takes a skilled and grown-up maternity department to handle this appropriately. It is all too easy to blame. Blame is not the same as being accountable for mistakes. A blame culture engenders fear and a reluctance by individuals to take responsibility for their failings.

If an otherwise efficient and conscientious member of staff makes a mistake and something dreadful happens as a consequence, they will need to be helped to understand what led them to taking that course of action. They may need support to forgive themselves and to find a way of living with themselves. Additionally, they may need others to have faith in their ability to be a good health worker. Unfortunately mistakes in medicine can have dreadful outcomes, especially in obstetrics, but it is essential that we understand that it is through mistakes that we often learn the most valuable lessons.

Sometimes the public will want staff that they hold responsible for the death or disability of their baby to be sacked. Unless gross negligence was involved then it is unlikely that this will happen. It is more likely that extra training or a period of supervised work would be arranged. It is, however, hugely important that parents and their wider family know that there are consequences of a mistake or mistakes having been made. This is not the same as condemning the staff member or members to becoming pariahs. Colleagues might do well to remember that 'there but for the grace of God go I'.

In our opinion, if we are honest, we have all made mistakes and sometimes will have got away with them – nothing serious happened or nobody else knew. At other times there will be investigations which call our actions into question and it is terribly important that the organisation is able to find a way to manage this so that a blame culture does not exist.

It is not unusual that patients complain when bad or difficult things happen as a result of being in hospital. Most of the time people's motivation for complaining includes the fact that they do not want anyone else to suffer as they have done. Additionally, they want a genuine and sincere apology for the mistakes that were made. This is an important lesson for Trusts to learn.

Trauma for staff – an obstetrician's view

My first boss and mentor, Jim Pearson, used to say 'If you haven't made a mistake then you're not working hard enough'. This is a mantra I have repeated countless times to numerous junior colleagues, to reassure them that everyone makes mistakes: the trick is to learn from them. Ideally you should try to learn from other people's mistakes as well as your own, but making a mistake in the first place does not make you a bad doctor or a bad person.

Fast forward from my first senior house officer (SHO) job to my first registrar job. I was in theatre removing someone's ruptured ectopic pregnancy, and the affected tube was a bit stuck to some of the pelvic wall at the back. The next day my consultant rang and asked me to meet him in the radiology department. It turned out that the specimen I'd sent to the lab had contained a tiny piece of the woman's ureter along with the ruptured fallopian tube, and an X-ray of her urinary tract had shown the site of the damage. My consultant and his friend, the senior radiologist, were standing next to the X-ray screen where my sin was on display, and they were both scowling at me. I felt awful. The patient was by now back in theatre where the urologists were fixing her ureter. The next morning I went to the urology ward to see her and to apologise for the damage and pain I'd caused. She looked at me and said 'you don't have to apologise – if it wasn't for you I would have died of a ruptured ectopic pregnancy. Thank you for saving my life'. It was then that I learnt that saying sorry is one of the most profoundly important things you can do when things go wrong – it isn't the terrifying and potentially inflammatory task that many of us were brought up during our training to believe that it might be. I later learnt that the patient had retroperitoneal fibrosis, and practically anyone dealing with her tube would have ended up damaging her ureter – it wasn't just down to me being incompetent, which is of course what I had originally decided. My internal critic was pretty insistent even then.

On another occasion, in the same hospital, I was the registrar on call on the labour ward. The consultant on call was at home. I was expected to get on with anything straightforward, but some situations were judged to be too complex for me to handle on my own, in which case the consultant would come in to help. A woman on the antenatal ward with a known major placenta praevia started bleeding at 35 weeks' gestation. She needed an emergency CS but when I phoned the boss he told me not to start the operation until he'd arrived. I did what he said and waited: the woman lost a huge amount of blood and the baby died. I was furious with myself for not disobeying the boss (but I was scared about what would happen if I did – I might have made an already dangerous situation worse), I was furious with my boss for not letting me start (I knew he was right in principle, but I thought he might have bent the rules), I was furious with Mother Nature for making the woman start to bleed at that moment. It still rankles thinking about it now, 35 or so years later.

Since those early days I have been involved with many cases where things have gone wrong and I've learnt that sometimes however hard I try, bad things will happen. Many patients understand this intuitively and do not apportion blame to any of the doctors or midwives who looked after them, but that generosity of spirit does not stop most of us feeling we are at fault. Our internal critic grumbles loudly and complains that we are not good enough.

Bad things happen and it's your fault

Years ago I was doing an elective CS list and one of the patients had opted to have a tubal ligation. It wasn't until I saw her the next day on the post-op round that I remembered that I hadn't tied her tubes. I apologised profusely and made arrangements for her to have a laparoscopic sterilisation on my elective gynaecology list six weeks later. She was very forgiving about my error but I learnt my lesson and vowed that I would never do it again. These days, with the WHO theatre checklist, everyone in the operating theatre knows what operation you're planning, but I still ask the theatre staff to keep an eye on me and remind me if they think I might forget to do what I'm supposed to do.

Bad things happen and it's someone else's fault

Again, many years ago, I was the consultant on call when the registrar took a woman to theatre for a second stage CS, and asked the midwife to push the baby's head up the pelvis to help the delivery of the head through the CS incision. The baby sustained a skull fracture as a result. This happened at a time when pushing up the baby's head was fairly common practice, and so criticism of the registrar by some of my colleagues seemed harsh, but nonetheless the skull fracture shouldn't have happened and our departmental recommendations for what you do in this situation changed as a result of this case.

Bad things happen and they could have been pre-empted and avoided

We looked after a couple who had a post-term stillbirth having declined offers to have labour induced. They were clear that they wanted to wait for labour to start naturally.

Unfortunately, by the time it did, it was 42 weeks and 4 days and the baby had died. This was an appalling thing to happen: many women go to 42 weeks and 4 days and beyond with no harm to the baby, but this family was not so lucky, and the fact that they had repeatedly declined induction just seemed to twist the knife.

The impact of this case on the staff was profound. At the debrief session that we arranged for the team, most of them were searching their memories to recall exactly what they had said to the couple and trying to figure out how they might have chosen their words in a way that would have made a difference: 'If only I'd expressed myself better/ more clearly/more firmly, maybe they would have changed their minds and the baby would have survived'. Looking around for someone to blame, they blamed themselves, internal critics chattering away constantly. Trying to make sense when something goes wrong is normal: the internal critic does this job by questioning what people did that could possibly have changed the outcome, even if, in fact, there wasn't anything else that they could have done.

During the debrief session, a few members of the team expressed anger with the parents for thinking that they knew best. They said that they wouldn't ever be able to face the couple and talk to them again, knowing that I would shortly have to do so in the perinatal loss clinic. I gently tried to point out that however hurt and angry we were all feeling, this amounted to nothing in comparison with the utter devastation the couple would be experiencing as a result of losing their child. They may have been doing similar kinds of questioning of their own motives and thinking 'if only we had listened to what we were told'. Equally, they may have been thinking that the policy wasn't made clear enough, putting the onus back on the staff rather than themselves.

Bad things happen and it's nobody's fault, not even yours, even though you are blamed

I know someone who witnessed a severe shoulder dystocia in which the baby sadly died. Not long afterwards he gave up obstetrics and switched to another specialty. In some ways this was a real shame, but it was completely understandable. Even if it wasn't your fault, you'd feel as if it was, and in any case it would be only natural to want to protect yourself against the chance of ever being hurt in that way again. You have to ask yourself whether the joy and satisfaction that you derive from your work is sufficient to make up for the crushing hurt and guilt you feel when things go badly wrong. For many of us, the joys thankfully outweigh the terrible sorrows, but this is not going to be the case for everyone.

To take another example, what if there is an emergency, which your senior registrar is dealing with to the best of his abilities, and at the same time you are in the midst of an operation because of an acute problem in a complex patient? Your complex patient does well but your senior registrar's patient has a catastrophe: the latter isn't really your fault, because you were in a different operating theatre, and you couldn't be in two places at once, but you were the consultant on call. You must shoulder the responsibility and you are the one criticised in the subsequent SI investigation report.

Criticism in a situation like this really stings. You had been presented with a choice, and you made a sensible decision: there are two patients needing help, and one is much more complex than the other, so of course you took the complex case whilst your very competent senior registrar took the other. It would definitely have been wrong and irresponsible to have allocated the cases differently, with you taking the 'easier' case and making your senior registrar deal with the complex one. You could not have foreseen what was about to happen, although later in your head you turn back the clock countless times and try to figure out how there might have been a better outcome. Of course you can't figure it out, and the more you try to square this circle, the more troubled you become. Your internal critic tells you loudly and forcefully that you're a bad person, that everything went wrong because of you, and if only one of your colleagues had been on duty instead of you everything would have been okay. This is of course nonsense, but that's not what you believe.

Being responsible

When you are the consultant on call, you are responsible for what goes on in your department. When one of your juniors does something that leads to a clinical incident, and you were in another room doing something else with another patient, whatever it was that happened is still your responsibility. You have to be the grown-up in this situation. You have to accept that whatever it was that your trainee did, they did it on your watch, and it is up to you to apologise to the patient, to make sure your trainee is not in a crumpled heap somewhere, and to continue to manage the unit efficiently so that everything else goes according to plan until the end of your shift.

As the trainee who has been directly involved in a serious incident, you need to assess quickly whether you are capable of continuing to work for the remainder of your shift, or whether you would be too much of a liability if you were to carry on. As soon as you can, you should take a copy of the relevant notes and CTGs, and record the times of the important aspects of the case, so that you can write a draft of your statement as soon as possible. This makes your statement more or less contemporaneous and consequently very credible when the people from the risk office request it.

As a consultant you have a responsibility to help your trainees when something has gone wrong, and to teach then firstly what to do in practical terms (make sure the correct clinical care is happening for both the patient concerned and anyone else on the unit, get the facts together to write a statement for the SI report) and secondly to help them learn about how they might handle the situation differently in the future. Most will feel guilty and upset, which is when the Jim Pearson mantra quoted earlier about everybody making mistakes comes into play.

Some junior staff may feel very wary of approaching a similar situation in the future, and may need a great deal of encouragement to do so. There is an element here of 'getting back on the bike'. Say for example one of your juniors accidentally cut a baby's skin whilst opening the uterus at a CS. You should offer to be their assistant the next time they do a CS, reassuring then that they can do the operation perfectly well and resisting the urge to take over and do it yourself.

The effect of trauma

There is a range of physical and psychological effects that accompany serious professional criticism. There are typical anxiety symptoms, including irritability, sudden tearfulness and sleep disturbance, which then of course messes up your ability to function the following day. Everything is much worse in the middle of the night: you wake up in a panic, going over what happened, trying to rewind the clock to change it but being unable to do so. You can become overly cautious about everything you try to do for fear of getting something else wrong. You are especially wary of doing anything complicated even though you would normally be perfectly capable of doing whatever it was. At the same time you feel as though you can't trust anyone else to do it either, so you are in a bind: you're afraid of doing it, but you're probably more afraid of letting someone else do it.

As well as the internal effects on you personally and the way in which you function, you can become very impatient with those close to you, who may not really understand what all the fuss is about and who might think they will make you feel better by trying to play it down. Any well-meaning friend saying 'don't worry, it'll all be fine' will be brusquely dismissed as being trite and stupid. We have written previously about the use-lessness of telling anyone not to worry; these incidents should indicate to a well-meaning friend that you might need to talk or be given time or a shoulder to cry on.

Your mind is taken over with worrying about what might happen. What if you end up being struck off? What would that mean? You've done nothing but medicine for many years, so what other work could you do? As well as the financial consequences of this possibility, the point that eats away at your brain is the potential loss of who you are. Of course you are a person first and a doctor second, but for so many years being a doctor has been a *very* close second, and the potential loss of that sense of self is mind-numbingly scary.

What helps? Time will gradually pass and you may be able eventually to see the events that troubled you so much in a new light. That said, you should be prepared for them to leave a lasting impression. This may take the form of learning from the experience and, in so doing, changing the practice for the better. The change might entail something fairly drastic, like my former professor who wouldn't let any of us learn to use a Ventouse; or something a little more subtle, like making a promise to yourself that (for example) you won't leave the labour ward until you know for certain that the Jehovah's Witness has suc-cessfully delivered her placenta without having a major haemorrhage.

Other people help, especially those who have been through something similar them-selves (and in obstetrics, there's almost always someone else who has). They can listen to you talk, rant or cry, and they can share their knowledge and experience so that you don't feel that you're the only one who has ever been in this position.

Hospital support systems work, if they exist, although sadly this was not always the case. It certainly was not the case in the past when one was expected to just 'get on with it'. These days, thankfully, there is a much greater understanding of the need for staff support and there are mechanisms that enable it to happen in a kind and constructive manner.

Work helps: you're almost certainly very good at what you do, and you should carry on doing it. The next case you manage successfully, the next operation you do that goes without a hitch, the next baby you deliver who obligingly cries immediately – all these things underline the fact that you're a competent professional and not a blundering liabil-ity. All these things muzzle the internal critic, at least for a while.

One way of separating from the internal critic is to realise that it is obsessed with being critical and completely ignores all of the positive aspects of your achievements. It is worth consciously silencing the critic by bringing in a balance and acknowledging yourself as a fine human being who is able to do all kinds of worthwhile things – something the critic knows nothing about. This is not easy for someone with a strong internal critic, but it is so important if we are to be as kind to ourselves as we are to those we meet in the course of our work.

Index

Printed in the United States
By Bookmasters